MY MOTHER SAID . . .

Reports of the Institute for Social Studies in Medical Care

The Institute for Social Studies in Medical Care was formed in 1970 as a development from the Institute of Community Studies, and its inauguration coincided with the publication by its Director Dr Ann Cartwright of *Parents and Family Planning Services*.

Further reports from the Institute for Social Studies in Medical Care will appear in this new series.

Medicine Takers, Prescribers and Hoarders
Karen Dunnell and Ann Cartwright

Life before Death
Ann Cartwright, Lisbeth Hockey and John L. Anderson

How many Children?
Ann Cartwright

A catalogue of series of Social Science books published by Routledge & Kegan Paul will be found at the end of this volume.

MY MOTHER SAID...

The way young people learned about sex and birth control

CHRISTINE FARRELL
in collaboration with
LEONIE KELLAHER

ROUTLEDGE & KEGAN PAUL
LONDON, HENLEY AND BOSTON

First published in 1978
by Routledge & Kegan Paul Ltd
39 Store Street,
London WC1E 7DD,
Broadway House,
Newtown Road,
Henley-on-Thames,
Oxon RG9 1EN and
9 Park Street,
Boston, Mass, 02108, USA
Printed in Great Britain by
Redwood Burn Limited
Trowbridge & Esher
© Christine Farrell 1978
No part of this book may be reproduced in
any form without permission from the
publisher, except for the quotation of brief
passages in criticism
British Library Cataloguing in Publication Data

Farrell, Christine
My mother said. – (Institute for Social
Studies in Medical Care; Reports).
1. Sex instruction – Great Britain
I. Title II. Series III. Kellaher, Leonie
616.6'007   HQ 56   78-40118

ISBN 0 7100 8850 7

My mother said that
I never should . . .
And my father said that
If I ever did,
He'd hit me on the head
With the teapot lid.

CONTENTS

Contents

Contents

ACKNOWLEDGMENTS

Many people have helped and contributed to this study:
The Department of Health and Social Security, who financed
it.
The young people and parents who gave up their time to
answer the questions.
The 52 interviewers who worked on the study, particularly
Margaret Anderson, Peter Bastick, Andrew Friend and Mike
McCabe, who were involved in other stages of its develop-
ment, and Mike Bennett and Charles Warwood who followed
up the more difficult final interviews.
The coders.
Ann Cartwright, who gave advice, support and encouragement
throughout.
Professor Alwyn Smith and members of the Department of
Community Medicine at Manchester University, who provided
accommodation and administrative help with training
sessions.
Sheila Grey, who helped us sort out sampling problems.
Rose Knight, who helped with national medical services
data.
Alison Britton, Suzan Gomez, Ann Pentol and Liz Smith,
who helped with tabulations and preparations.
Barbara Edwards who typed the questionnaires, and Janet
Ball who typed the report.
Members of the Institute's Advisory Committee: Abe
Adelstein, Tony Alment, Valerie Beral, Leslie Best, Bill
Brass, Vera Carstairs, May Clarke, John Fry, Spence
Galbraith, Geoffrey Hawthorn, Austin Heady (Chairman),
Margot Jefferys, Joyce Leeson, John McEwan, David Morrell,
Martin Richards, Alan Snaith, Michael Warren.
The Department of Education and Science who financed a six-
week pilot study of teachers' attitudes to sex education.
Maureen O'Brien, Simon Stander and Warwick Wilkins all
gave support, encouragement and ideas, and Alison Smith
had the difficult task of checking the final draft.

1

INTRODUCTION

This is a study of the sources of information young people
encountered during their early years, which helped them
(or hindered them) in the acquisition of knowledge about
sex and birth control. It describes how young people in
the 1970s remembered learning about sex, and illustrates
some of the problems they met. In this way, whilst
exploring the nature of their sources of information and
the relationship these have to their attitudes to sex and
contraception, it becomes possible to suggest ways in
which the transmission of such information can be improved.
   The study also looks at the sexual behaviour of
adolescents, because contraceptive knowledge and practice
are obviously closely related to sexual knowledge and
practice. Without sex, contraception is irrelevant.
Schofield's study of teenage sexual behaviour suggested
that a fifth of the boys and an eighth of the girls in his
survey had engaged in full sexual intercourse (Schofield,
1965, p.40). In a more recent study of female students at
Aberdeen University, 44% said they were sexually experienced (McCance and Hall, 1972). Although there are no
more recent data than Schofield's (collected in the early
1960s) about the proportion of young unmarried people
having intercourse, it would seem reasonable to assume
(if it is true that our society has become increasingly
permissive) that the proportion of young people 'at risk'
of unwanted pregnancy has increased. The media frequently
assure us that young people are more 'permissive' than
they were ten years ago. The evidence available, of
increasing numbers of conceptions to single girls in the
under 20 age group, when this study was first conceived,
suggested that this might be true. Between 1962 and 1972,
illegitimate births to women under 20 years as a percentage
of all live births to the age group increased from 20.7%
to 27.5%. The number of legal abortions for this age group

1

increased between 1969 and 1974 from 9,230 to 27,040.
Figures since then and since this study was completed
show that this rate of increase for abortions has
declined, and the illegitimacy and premarital conception
rates are beginning to fall. The numbers, however, are
still high and the reasons for the increase during the
past ten years need to be explored.

Two of the reasons often given for the alleged increase
in sexual activity amongst teenagers are the availability
of the pill and the Abortion Act. The first, the most
effective method of preventing pregnancy yet discovered
(setting aside sterilisation which is not for young
people), the second the now legal way to solve the problem
of unwanted pregnancies. As the number of abortions
carried out on young unmarried girls increased at a time
when there was a very effective method of contraception
available, it seemed important to explore the reasons why.
One explanation is that the rise in the number of legal
abortions since 1969 only reflects the availability of a
service. But there are people who believe that the
availability of abortion encourages premarital sex.

It seems likely that early sources of information about
sex and birth control may determine practice, effective or
otherwise, during adulthood. In her study 'Family Planning
Services in England and Wales', Bone (1973) concluded that
to be most effective services should 'seek to avert premarital conceptions'. But, as she herself admitted, her
enquiry only described the situation as it was and could
not seriously attempt to explain why. By studying a group
of young people who are at, or close to, the stage of
learning about sex and birth control and also at an age
where they might become premaritally pregnant, it should
be possible to attempt more of an explanation of why those
who fail to avoid unwanted pregnancies do so.

But the study is not solely concerned with young people
who are sexually active and the reasons for their use or
non-use of birth-control methods. It is also concerned
with other young people who are not sexually active and
may not become so until after they are married. They also
are at risk to unwanted pregnancies if they marry and do
not know how to plan their families. During the 1950s and
1960s there was a continuous increase in the numbers of
young people marrying in their teens and a peak was
reached in 1970 after the legal age of marriage without
parental consent was lowered to 18. In 1970 the marriage
rate for 16 to 19-year-old girls was 95.4 and for boys in
the same age group it was 27.2. Since then the rates
have fallen consistently, until in 1975 they returned
almost to the level of the early 1960s (78.1 for girls

and 21.5 for boys) (Office of Population Censuses and
Surveys, 1975, Table 23). The number of births to married
teenagers has also fallen during the 1970s and there is
some evidence that young married couples are delaying the
birth of their first child (Cartwright, 1976, pp.7-10;
Pearce, 1975, pp.6-8). As Thompson points out, the fact
that the number of abortions for married women has remained
fairly constant since 1972 and the number of births to the
same group has declined implies 'that contraceptive
practice has become more effective and this is consistent
with what we know about motivations; the tendency of
younger married couples to delay the start of childbearing
as well as the shift to smaller family size as compared
with, say, a decade ago' (Thompson, 1976, pp.3-8). If
this is true and the recent levelling out of the number of
premarital conceptions has the same explanation, this study
should help to establish that fact and also attempt to
explain why some young people are using contraception
effectively whilst others are not.

The availability of and publicity given to birth-control
services and contraceptive methods, particularly the pill,
have certainly increased during the last decade. Some
girls who took part in the study expressed the feeling
that they should be 'on the pill' even though they were not
sexually active, 'just in case'. Whilst this shows
admirable forethought it is also a symptom of the kinds of
pressures that teenage girls are subject to, often unnecessarily. The publicity given to the increase in the
number of abortions and the numbers of schoolgirl mothers
is not always accompanied by a full discussion of the
availability and suitability of birth-control methods for
teenagers. Although clinic and general practitioner
services are now available to teenagers, they themselves
may not know of them or regard them as freely accessible.
Also, whilst the pill is the most effective reversible
method of contraception, it is not always the most
appropriate method for some patterns of sexual activity.
One of the aims of this study was therefore to look at
the ways in which young people are prepared for sexual
activity and to assess how relevant this preparation was
for their current and future needs.

In talking to doctors and educators about sex education
for young people, it seemed that most of them felt that
parents were the 'ideal' first source of information.
But little is known about how parents themselves feel
about telling their children or how effective they are as
a source of information. What evidence there is suggests
that there is a strong class bias in whether and how
parents discuss sexual topics. The Newsons' study of

child-rearing patterns in Nottingham (1968, p.454)
pointed to the different ways in which middle-class and
working-class parents talked to their children. In
'Parents and Family Planning Services' (Cartwright, 1970,
p.210) it was shown that working-class mothers more often
used the less effective methods of birth control and had
more unintended pregnancies. Also the mother's level of
education was an important determinant of whether
professional advice about birth control was sought. It
seems likely therefore that many parents would not be,
or would not feel, capable of giving their children the
information they would need to deal with their involvement in a sexual relationship. Because parents are an
important potential source of information about sexual
matters, and since it was proposed to ask young people
what kinds of information they had received from their
parents, a secondary aim of the study was to explore
parental views on the subject. By asking mothers and
fathers whom they felt should tell their children about
sex and birth control and what kinds of information they
had given their own children, it was possible to look at
the ways in which parents regarded themselves as
information-providers.

Traditionally, believing sex education to be the
province of parents, schools have been reluctant to
become involved in anything but the presentation of the
basic biological 'facts'. As Dallas (1972) points out in
her book 'Sex Education in School and Society', 'Facts
were enough and sex was put over in a way similar to
that used when dealing with the maps of the coalfields.
The only difference was the special atmosphere which
surrounded the short, sharp talk. It must often have
conveyed to its victims that these matters were unspeak-
able and that no well-bred pupil would either need or
dare to investigate them further.' She goes on to say
that this method of sex education had one advantage, 'it
did not attract unfavourable criticism from parents or
education committees, largely because all concerned were
much too embarrassed to mention it'.

Fortunately sex education in schools has, in many
areas, evolved beyond this stage. Research and determined
effort has produced sex-education programmes of high
quality like the Nuffield Secondary Science Project and
the Schools Council Moral Education Project. But still
in many schools no such programmes exist and adolescents
have to rely on one or two 'short, sharp talks' for their
information. And some do not even have that. There is
no comprehensive review of sex education in schools, but
it seems to be largely a matter of luck and teachers'

inclinations whether young people are taught about sex and birth control at school. Half of the boys in Schofield's study of teenage sexual behaviour and one-seventh of the girls said they had not received any sex education lessons at school. Sixteen per cent of the boys in his sample and 18% of the girls knew nothing about birth control and 'many of the others had only a slight knowledge of contraceptives'. However, Schofield's study was completed over ten years ago, and many things have changed during this period. Another of the aims of this study was to look at the ways in which young people are told about sex and birth control at school and how adequate they felt this information was in terms of their present and future needs.

The peer group is known to be a major source of information on sexual matters for teenagers. Gagnon and Simon (1973) point out in their book 'Sexual Conduct' that in American studies the fact that 'the primary source of sex information is the peer group has been a stable characteristic of most of the populations studied, beginning with the Max Exner study of 1915.' In Britain there is evidence from the Schofield study that friends are the most common source of information and also that premarital sexual behaviour is influenced by peer group attachments (1965, Chapter 10). It seems evident that friends are an important source of information, but the way in which they influence attitudes and behaviour has not been fully explored. This is also one of the areas considered in the study.

There are a number of other possible sources of information, including books, films, television, magazines and newspapers, from which children almost certainly acquire information. These sources were not explored as fully as the others, for two reasons. During the pre-pilot and pilot stages of the study, when less structured questions were asked, parents, teachers and friends emerged clearly as the predominant sources recollected by the young people. At the pilot stage they themselves seemed to suggest that they considered 'media' sources subsidiary or complementary to the three 'human' sources. The other reason was the difficulty experienced by the young people in recollecting from which books, films or magazines they had acquired information and at which stages. It is possible that by concentrating attention and questions on parents, teachers and friends their importance has been over-emphasised; on the other hand, it was clear that this reflected the way the teenagers recollected their sources.

Professional advisers may also be used as sources of

information, particularly when knowledge of birth control
is required. But as far as is known, there are no studies
which provide evidence on the extent to which doctors or
para-medical workers contribute to the learning process.
This study looks at their role as information providers
both within schools and within their own clinics and
surgeries.

Historical evidence on the way information about sex
was learned or transmitted suggests that children and
young adults, particularly girls, were told nothing at all
or very little and were expected to become acquainted with
the 'facts' only after they were married. Crow (1971)
quotes from a Victorian source, 'Memories Discreet and
Indiscreet' by Mrs Menzies, an account of her almost total
ignorance of sex when she married. And many autobiogra-
phies and biographies of women who grew up during the
late Victorian, early twentieth-century period offer
insights into sexual ignorance (e.g., Bell, 'Virginia
Woolf'; McCarthy in 'Memories of a Catholic Girlhood'; and
O'Brien in 'Country Girls'). These experiences may not be
typical, but they do suggest that sex was often an un-
mentionable and frightening subject. Seymour-Smith
suggests that Victorian morality is the basis for
twentieth-century attitudes to sex and says, in his book
'Sex and Society' (1975), 'A survey of sex in the 20th
century would be impossible without a preliminary look at
the sexual mores and practices of the century that
precedes it and from which it arose, ... our society is
more subject to Victorian sexual attitudes - especially
in its reactions to them - than it imagines.' Although
there is undoubtedly a great deal more openness today
about sexuality than there has been during the past 100
years, it is still generally true to say, as did two
American authors recently, that 'learning about sex in
our society is learning about guilt; conversely learning
how to manage sexuality constitutes learning how to
manage guilt' (Gagnon and Simon, 1973, p.42).

The problems for researchers wanting to explore a
learning process in any area are severe. In an area like
sex and birth control where young people are involved in
learning not only factual information about their own
bodies but also in dealing with their own emotional
reactions and social customs and taboos, the problems
become even more difficult. The process of learning
about sex and sexual relationships is not only a matter
of receiving information, having it reinforced and
finally assimilating it, but is complicated by the need
to learn how to deal with strong emotional feelings and
how to cope with physical desires, to say nothing of

learning to deal with the social implications of
behaviour. Such a complex and lengthy process could not
be covered in a survey like this. To explore the assimi-
lation of sexual knowledge and the psycho-sexual processes
involved would need an in depth study over a long period.
The main aim of this study was therefore to explore the
primary sources of information on sex and birth control
for young people and the relationship, if there is one,
between their sources of information, their attitudes to
sex and birth control, and their sexual and contraceptive
behaviour.

METHODS

It is widely acknowledged that the location of a sample
of teenagers on a random basis is difficult. They are a
mobile group and there are no comprehensive lists from
which they can be selected. Schofield outlines some of
the problems in his study, and he himself failed to get
a random sample, although he felt that his teenagers
were representative of their age group (1965, pp.13-21
and pp.276-83). The main criticism of Schofield's
methodology is that the seven areas used were not randomly selected nor were they selected on the same basis. He
also used different sampling frames in the different
areas. In one area the Executive Council's list was
used; in two other areas, school attendance lists; and
in the four remaining areas a market research agency
called on all the houses in selected districts to locate
the teenagers. Other studies of young people have
usually drawn their samples from either local or special
groups (e.g. Gill, Illsley and Koplik, 1970; Willmott,
1966; Davies and Stacey, 1972). Given the nature of the
study and the fact that at the time it was initiated
there was a worrying rise in the number of teenage
abortions and pregnancies, it seemed important that a
national random sample should be used.

Areas

The study was carried out in 12 areas of England and
Wales between July 1974 and January 1975. The areas
chosen were local authority metropolitan and non-metropolitan districts and were selected with probability
proportional to population. Equal numbers of addresses
in each area were selected from the electoral registers
so that everyone had the same chance of being included.

This initial stage of selecting addresses was necessary
to identify the places where young people lived. (A list
of the areas and their population size is given in
Appendix I with a full description of the methods used.)
A letter explaining the nature of the study and asking if
anyone aged 16 to 19 lived there was sent to a named
person at each address, together with a returnable form.

Sample Size

To achieve a completed sample of approximately 1,500
young people (this number was required because it would
allow cross-analysis and was small enough to be manage-
able) a sample of 1,604 addresses was selected at random
from the electoral registers in each area. Table 1 shows
the response to this postal screen.

TABLE 1   Response to postal screen

	%
Responded:	
Had young person aged 16-19	9.6
Did not have young person aged 16-19	68.1
Total replied	77.7
Wrote refusing to say	1.2
Informed house void/occupant dead	0.9
No response	20.2
Number of addresses written to (= 100%)	19,224

RESPONSE TO THE POSTAL SCREEN AND INTERVIEW APPROACH

The 19,224 letters produced 1,840 addresses at which at
least one young person aged between 16 and 19 was said to
live. Interviewers were briefed to call at these
addresses and interview all the young people in the age
group who lived there. A preliminary identification
stage was necessary, because the initial form had asked
only for the sex of young people and whether they lived
permanently at that address. Interviewers therefore used
an initial approach sheet to record the names, sex and
dates of birth of all young people at each address. In
practice it often proved difficult for interviewers to
get all this information if a respondent was determined
to refuse. But in all cases it was possible to establish

how many young people lived at each address and whether
they were male or female.   Table 2 shows the number of
addresses from which positive replies were received, the
number of addresses providing wrong information, and the
total number of young people 'found' from these addresses.

TABLE 2   Number of addresses and young people produced by
the postal screen

	All areas
Number of addresses saying 'yes' in response to initial letter	1,840
Number of addresses providing wrong information (i.e. no young people)	114
Total 'correct' addresses	1,726
Total number of young people living at correct addresses	2,110
Average number of young people at each address	1.22

The number of addresses giving positive replies and the
numbers of young people located in this way varied from
area to area.   The area with the largest number of young
people was Merseyside with 221, and the area yielding the
smallest number was Devon with 148.

INTERVIEW RESPONSE

The response to a request for an interview with the 2,110
young people found through the postal screen was 74%.
This is lower than rates achieved in some other studies
of young people but higher than Schofield achieved.
Willmott (1966) had an 88% response and Sirey and Power
(1974) had a 77% response.   Both these studies were East
End studies which may account for some of the difference.
They were also both studies of boys whereas our sample
was mixed.   The National Children's Bureau cohort study
of 16-year-olds obtained some data from 79.5% of its
sample.   But again this study is different because of its
longitudinal nature (Fogelman, 1976).   Schofield's
interview response rate was 66% but the difference was
not due to a higher refusal rate (Schofield's was 12%
compared with our 16%), but to the number of young people
he was unable to interview (22% to our 10%) (1965,
pp.296-302).   Altogether 346 teenagers refused to take

part in this study, and approximately one in every three
refusals came from the parents before the young person
had been approached. Just under a third were indirect
refusals (classified as such if the young person consistently broke appointments or generally evaded the interviewer) either by parents or young people, and just over
a third were direct refusals from the teenagers. The
reasons they gave for refusing were mainly apathy, not
wanting to be bothered or not having time.

The reasons why the remaining 208 young people were
not available for interview varied from being away at sea,
away at college or working away from home.

TABLE 3   Response to interview approach

	All areas %
Completed interviews	74
Refusals	16
Not available for interview	10
Number of young people (= 100%)	2,110
Number of addresses approached	1,840

The response rate within the different areas varied from
81% in Merseyside to 64% in Devon. This should not be
taken as evidence of the greater interest in sex in
Liverpool and a lack of interest in Devon. The reasons
for such a wide variation are probably more related to
the persistence of the interviewers and the proportions
of young people living at home than anything else.
Variations in the proportions being interviewed, refusing
and unavailable by area are given in Appendix I.

If the response is calculated from both stages of the
sample an overall rate of 57% was achieved. Because the
original sample was of addresses and the total number of
young people at these addresses was unknown, this figure
has been calculated by assuming that similar proportions
of young people were in the original sample and the group
who co-operated. It is not unusual to have rates as low
as this. For example, Sorenson (1973) approached a
random sample of 839 young people (from 2,042 households
located by a market research agency). Of these 839, 47%
(393) were interviewed. It does mean, however, that
biases in the sample are inevitable. The possibility of
investigating the nature of these biases was considered
but rejected for a number of financial and public relations
reasons, discussed in more detail in Appendix I.

THE INTERVIEWERS

Because this study included questions in the sensitive area of sexual and contraceptive behaviour, it seemed appropriate to use interviewers who were near to the ages of the young people being interviewed. Schofield emphasised the importance of using young interviewers and it is obvious that teenagers would not always feel comfortable talking about such things to people similar in age to their parents. The average age of our interviewers was 23. Schofield also stressed the need to use male interviewers for male respondents and female interviewers for female respondents (1965, p.20 and private communication). Although there is little evidence on this question of using the same sex interviewers (Cartwright and Moffett, 1974) it seemed advisable not to risk embarrassment on either side. Thus two male and two female interviewers were recruited to work in each area. They were mainly students, teachers or social work students.

THE INTERVIEWS

The first part of the interview dealt with questions of relationships with parents, work, educational experience, leisure activities and peer group friendships and activities. The teenagers were then asked about the way they had first learned about reproduction, sexual intercourse and birth control. Three sets of questions followed which dealt in turn with the three sources of information, parents, school and peer group. Questions about methods of birth control came next and then questions about their own sexual experience. Finally they were asked about their parents' education, religion and occupations and the composition of the family. The majority of interviews (71%) lasted between one and two hours, 19% took between half an hour and one hour, and 10% lasted for over two hours. Almost all the interviews were carried out without anyone else in the room (93%).

The question always asked in a survey involving personal and sensitive areas is 'How do you know they are telling the truth?' The honest answer is that we do not. Truth tests can and have been devised and there are methods of reducing the opportunities for respondents to give false answers (see Belson, 1975 for details of attempts to do this). Tests like these were not used partly because the interview was already long, but primarily because such scales (for example, the Crown Marlow Socially Desirable

Scale) only test consistency and do not necessarily mean
that other questions have been answered truthfully. Apart
from designing the questions to minimise opportunities
for fantasy, it seems that the most important factor in
gathering 'facts' and opinion by interview and questionnaire is the skill of the interviewer in establishing a
relationship with the respondent.

Another problem was the presence of parents in the
house during the interview. Although interviewers were
instructed to conduct the interview in private and never
to interview with someone else in the room, the risk of
parents popping in or passing through could be sufficient
to limit the fullness of answers to some questions. A
second interviewer interviewing the mother or father at
the same time did not always remove this risk, since the
other parent and siblings remained as potential intruders.
Short of interviewing the whole household there was
little to be done about this. The possibility of interviewing outside the home was considered, but because
addresses were not clustered a lot of travelling would
have been involved, or a great many rooms would have had
to have been hired. There is also the problem of
persuading the young people to come to an office. On
this question, the possible limited nature of the answers
to some questions has to be set against the possible loss
of a considerable number of interviews. All the interviewers agreed that in many cases, if the young people
were not interviewed at the first approach or soon after,
they became increasingly reluctant and more determined
to refuse.

THE INTERVIEWS WITH MOTHERS AND FATHERS

The sample of parents was drawn from the 1,840 positive
replies to the postal screen. One in every three of
these addresses was selected for a parent interview, and
every other one of these allocated to a mother or a
father. Only one parent was approached for interview at
each address.

The response rate is lower from the parents than from
the young people. Table 4 shows that nearly two-thirds
were interviewed (62%) compared with three-quarters of
the young people. This is partly due to the complicated
interview arrangements necessary at these addresses, and
partly because interviewers were told that if only one
person could be interviewed it should be the young person.

TABLE 4   Interview response for mothers and fathers

	Mothers	Fathers	All parents approached
	%	%	%
Interviewed	65	59	62
Refused	25	26	25
Unavailable for interview (because dead, separated, untraceable)	10	15	13
Number (= 100%)	288	277	565*

* 601 addresses were selected for parent interviews but 36 were addresses where respondents had given wrong information and so were excluded.

The interviews with the mothers and fathers were shorter than the young people's. Just over half (58%) took between one and two hours; a third (35%) took between half an hour and an hour, and the rest (7%) took two hours or more.

The parents were asked questions which dealt with the way they thought young people should learn about reproduction, sexual intercourse and birth control. These were followed by questions about the kinds of information they had given their own child, who was usually one of the young people interviewed (for details see Appendix III).

Altogether 1,905 people were interviewed: 1,556 teenagers, 186 mothers and 163 fathers.

THE TEENAGERS

Discussing and describing the general characteristics of a sample population can be a dull task. What was a number of interesting, widely varying individuals with different ideas, attitudes and experiences becomes a group statistic. But for two reasons it seems important to provide these data. First, the representative nature of the sample needs to be discussed, and second, it is useful for the reader to have a picture of the kinds of young people who took part in the study. Individual comments and experiences will be used later and it is hoped that this will help to bring the group statistics to life.

Sex

Half the teenagers were boys and half were girls. The
proportions were 50.3% boys and 49.7% girls. In 1971 the
Census proportions for 13 to 16-year-old boys and girls
were 51.5% and 48.5% respectively. (The group who were
16-19 in 1974 would have been 13-16 in 1971 at the time
of the Census.) The differences, whilst not statistically
significant, can be accounted for by the fact that more
boys than girls were lost from the initial sample.
Proportions of boys and girls in the 2,110 initial sample
were 51.1% and 48.9% respectively. This loss occurred
because more boys were unavailable for interview. The
refusal rate for boys and girls was similar.

Age

In the age group nationally, equal proportions are found
in the different year groups, that is a quarter are 16,
17, 18 and 19. In the study group 23% were 16, 26% were
17, 26% were 18 and 25% were 19. This difference arose
because the sample was selected in May 1974, but not
interviewed until after July - by which time some of the
16-year-olds had become 17. At the other end of the age
group, the 19-year-olds who had become 20 were still
interviewed and classified as 19.

Marital status

The majority of boys and girls were single (94%), although
this included 8% who said they were engaged to be married.
A small group (6%) were already married, and in spite of
some concern at the pilot stage that this was a group that
was likely to be under-represented in the sample, our
proportions were not significantly different from the
national figures. For boys the proportions were exactly
the same, 2% in the sample and 2% of all 16 to 19-year-
olds. For girls 8.7% of the sample were married compared
with 9.9% of all 16 to 19-year-old girls married in 1974
(Office of Population Censuses and Surveys' unpublished
estimates of marital status of 16-19-year-olds in England
and Wales at 30 June 1974). This slight under-representation of married girls (which was not statistically significant) may have arisen because some of the girls who were
unavailable for interview may have married and moved away
in between the time the sample was selected and the interviewers called at their address.

Work status

Nearly two-thirds of the teenagers were working (60%),
with 16% at school, 14% at college and a further 8% who
were unemployed;   2% gave their occupation as 'housewife'.
Comparisons with national figures are virtually impossible
because detailed age breakdowns are not published. The
only available figures (in suitable form) are the Department of Education and Science records of the numbers of
children in each age group who were attending school in
January in 1974. These are shown in detail in Appendix I.
There is a suggestion of a slight under-representation in
the sample of the number of 18-year-olds still at school.

Social class

An examination of the social class composition of the
sample group raises some problems. It is not sensible to
classify them on the basis of their own occupations
because so many of them were still at school or college.
Also the occupations of those who were working cannot be
said to reflect their ultimate classification. All social
class analysis has therefore been done on the basis of
father's occupation. Apart from the well recognised
difficulties of using the Registrar General's classification of occupations, other problems arise because their
occupations have been reported by sons and daughters.
There is some evidence that where parental occupations
are reported by children there is a tendency for them to
report slightly higher status jobs. However, this
tendency does not seem to affect the two main groups;
children of manual workers do not report their fathers'
occupations as non-manual or vice-versa (Niemi, 1974,
p.25). With this in mind, 38% of the young people in the
sample reported that their fathers had non-manual occupations, 55% said they had manual occupations, 2% said their
fathers were in the armed forces, and 5% of the replies
were unclassifiable. Since no national data are published
about the social class of fathers of children aged 16 to
19, no direct comparisons can be made. The most suitable
figures available are those in the 1971 Census under the
heading 'chief economic supporter of household' (Central
Statistical Office, 1974, Table 39). Here the proportions
were 34% non-manual, 53% manual and 13% unclassifiable.
This comparison, although unsatisfactory, indicates that
the relative proportions in each broad classification in
our sample are not greatly different from those in the
population.

Place of birth

The majority of teenagers said they had been born in the
British Isles (95%); 1% gave India and Pakistan as their
place of birth; 1% said the West Indies and 1% said
Africa. A further 1% named Cyprus, Malta, Gibraltar or
another European country, and the rest (1%) came from
other parts of the world. No age breakdown is available
for place of birth nationally, but for persons in Great
Britain aged 16 and over (Office of Population Censuses
and Surveys, 1973, Table 1.20) the proportions are 95%
born in the British Isles, 1% India, Pakistan, Ceylon and
Bangladesh, 1% Caribbean and 3% elsewhere. Where the
grouping of countries in the sample and the General
Household Survey coincide, agreement of the proportions
born in these countries is good. On several occasions it
was necessary to use interpreters for interviews with
parents and young people.

Where it has been possible to compare the characteristics
of the sample group with the proportions occurring in the
age group nationally or with the population as a whole,
the comparisons indicate that the young people in the
sample are representative of the age group. Having
demonstrated this, however, it is still true to say that
the young people interviewed were a collection of individuals who talked about their individual views, attitudes
and experiences. We cannot claim, therefore, that these
views and attitudes are representative of anything other
than the teenagers who took part in the study. Insofar
as they are a sub-sample of the age group they may be
said to reflect some patterns of behaviour and experiences.
With this in mind the structure of the book has been
organised to discuss these experiences and the learning
process.
    The first chapters deal with the sexual experience of
the young people interviewed and their use and knowledge
of birth control. Chapter 4 presents an overview of their
sources of information on reproduction, sexual intercourse
and birth control. Chapters 5, 6 and 7 concentrate on
learning within the family: first, what the teenagers
remembered their parents telling them, then parental
attitudes and actions, followed by a discussion of family
relationships and their influence on learning, attitudes
and behaviour. Chapters 8 and 9 deal with sex education
at school and relationships with teachers, and Chapters
10 and 11 with friends as a source of information and
peer group relationships. Teenage attitudes to and use
of doctors and birth control clinics are discussed in

Chapter 12, and the penultimate chapter looks at the
ways in which sexual activity and use of birth control
are related to the way in which young people learned
about sex and birth control and their satisfaction with
the way they learned. The final chapter contains a
summary and recommendations.

Statistical tests (e.g., t test, chi square, difference
of proportions and x^2 trend) have been applied throughout
to guard against attributing significance to variations
in data which could have occurred by chance. Only when
these tests revealed that differences and trends in the
figures had a probability of less than 0.05 of arising
by chance, has attention been drawn to them, unless
otherwise stated in the text.

2

SEXUAL BEHAVIOUR

Premarital sexual experience was classified by an
American sociologist as deviant behaviour as recently as
1970. Reiss (1970, pp.78-87) claimed that it qualified
as such 'on the basic ground that in the eyes of most
adults it is viewed as the violation of a norm, and many
people hold this view with sufficient intensity to place
such behaviour outside their tolerance limits.' Publicly
expressed disapproval of sex before marriage was put on
record by Britain as recently as 1975. The 'official'
attitude according to an International Planned Parenthood
Federation survey (1975) was given as approving only of
sex after marriage even though the most widespread
attitude in the country as a whole was given as approving
of sex before marriage if it grew from love for the other
person and 'even then only after a considerable time'.
   A double standard thus emerges which can be confusing
for young people. On the one hand they are told that sex
before marriage is wrong and on the other are constantly
made aware of 'sex' and its attractions through the media,
particularly through advertising. The newspapers throw
up their print in horror at the increasing number of
pregnant schoolgirls, on the page before they show full
frontal nudes.
   The system of controls over premarital sexual relationships has lessened over the past 50 years for a variety
of economic and social reasons. As Illsley and Taylor
(1974) point out,
   The strong taboo on premarital sexual relationships...
   has been heavily breached and indeed a counter-ideology
   condemning the taboo and associated sanctions has
   arisen based on notions of self-expression, warmth of
   human relationships and preparation for marriage. The
   new 'model' has of course been facilitated by the
   greater efficiency of contraceptive techniques, their

wider availability and by access to abortion in the
event of contraceptive failures.
So disapproval competes with a new philosophy of fulfilment and the resulting tension shows itself in the
uncertainty of the young.

This chapter looks at young people's attitudes to
premarital sex, and the teenage pattern of sexual experience and use of contraception, as a preliminary to
subsequent attempts to relate experience to the way in
which the young people said that they had learned about
sex and birth control.

ATTITUDES TO SEX BEFORE MARRIAGE

The attitudes of the young people in this study were
mainly in favour of sex before marriage. They were asked
'Do you have any views on sex before marriage? Could you
say whether you approve, disapprove or have mixed feelings
about it?' If they had mixed feelings they were asked
'Would you say you are more inclined to approve or disapprove or are you equally balanced?' Additional comments
were given (though not asked for) by 48%. Nearly half of
them said outright that they approved of it; less than
one in ten said they definitely disapproved, and the rest
said they had mixed feelings about the question. More of
those who had mixed feelings were inclined towards
approval than disapproval, but a fifth said they were
unable to sort out their feelings sufficiently to decide
whether they were inclined to approve or disapprove.
Girls were less likely to say they approved, but their
lack of approval was made up for by mixed feelings rather
than disapproval, as Table 5 shows.

TABLE 5   Attitudes to sex before marriage

	Male	Female	All
	%	%	%
Approve	60	37	49
Disapprove	7	10	8
Mixed feelings	32	52	42
Don't know/can't say	1	1	1
Number (= 100%)	779	771	1,550*

* 6 excluded because replies inadequate.

The people who disapproved gave a variety of reasons for
their disapproval. Some were religious:
   'It's contrary to the Bible ... because of the sacred
   state of marriage.'
Some were social:
   'Mainly I disapprove from what I've seen of people
   having to get married and the conditions they live in.'
   'Don't think it should be allowed because of over-
   population.'
Some were linked to personal experience:
   'Now I don't really believe in it because it doesn't
   work out. If you fall and have to get married as we
   did and it didn't work out. Since I've had the
   experience I feel it's worse on the woman really.'
   However, amongst those who expressed additional
comments to this question, the widespread view was that
premarital sex was acceptable if it happened as a result
of a stable relationship and care was taken to avoid
unwanted pregnancy:
   'I think sex before marriage is alright as long as you
   don't just sleep around with anyone. I think if you're
   going steady with someone for a long time - but just
   to sleep with anyone I think is wrong.'
   'I believe that when one feels one is mature enough to
   lead a healthy spiritual relationship then one is also
   mature enough to lead a healthy sex relationship if
   the right precautions are taken.'
The next most common view was that it was a decision which
should be left to the individuals concerned:
   'I think it's entirely up to the couple concerned, as
   long as they're sort of ... kids, that's ridiculous,
   12, 13, they're at it now, but the over-age couple
   they know what they're doing - if they don't they
   shouldn't be doing it.'
   Outright approval without qualification was not common
and some young people mentioned that they disapproved
strongly of sleeping around with anyone (9%):
   'Well, I think if you really do love a bloke I don't
   see why you should wait till you're married, but you
   have to be careful or you might end up sleeping around
   and that's not good.'
A few (4%) made the point spontaneously that sex before
marriage was necessary as a precaution against an unhappy
marriage:
   'It's nice to know what you're going to live with
   instead of waiting until you're married to know what
   the bloke's like. Even though it's against my religion,
   I think it's good because you know what you're going to
   live with.'

And more succinctly:
'You have to try your shoes on before you buy them.'
Two trends were suggested by the data: the first showed
the older age groups more likely to say they approved of
premarital sex (56% of 19-year-olds approved compared with
38% of 16-year-olds); the second suggests that middle-class
children are less likely to say they approve than working-
class teenagers. This can be explained by a movement to
greater congruence between attitudes and behaviour since
subsequent data show that 19-year-olds and boys from
working-class families are more likely to be sexually
experienced.

SEXUAL EXPERIENCE

In 1964, 16% of Schofield's sample of 15 to 19-year-olds
said that they had had sexual intercourse at least once.
In this sample of 16 to 19-year-olds, ten years later,
51% said they were sexually experienced, 45% said they
had not had any sexual experience and 4% refused to
answer the question ('Could you tell me if you have had
sexual intercourse?' If they said 'Yes' or were uncertain they were asked 'Does that mean you have "gone
all the way"?'). The comparison is not a clear one
because of the inclusion of the younger age group in the
1964 sample, but there has obviously been an increase in
the numbers of teenagers saying that they have had sexual
intercourse. The proportion of boys in the 1974 sample
who said they were experienced was 55% and the proportion
of girls 46%. This bears out Schofield's findings of ten
years ago, that boys become sexually experienced at an
earlier age than girls (20% of boys aged 15-19 and 12% of
girls in the same age group said they were sexually
experienced in 1964 (Schofield, 1965, pp.39-40)). If the
married young people are excluded from our sample, as they
were from Schofield's, 54% of all single males in the
sample said they were sexually experienced and 42% of the
single girls, an overall figure for unmarried teenagers
aged 16-19 of 48%.

Age of first sexual experience

Nearly half of those who said they were sexually experienced said that they had had their first experience
before they were 16. This means that a fifth (21%) of
the whole sample had had at least one sexual experience
by the time they were 16; three-quarters of them were boys.
Twelve per cent of all the girls in the sample said they
had had intercourse by that age and 31% of all the boys.

Although this is a question to which young people may be
tempted to give an exaggerated answer, the possibility that
over a third of all teenagers in the sample had had some
sexual experience before or by the age of 16 has important
implications for sex educationists and medical services
offering contraceptive advice. Table 6 shows the proportion
of boys and girls who said that they had had sexual intercourse by their current age and the age they were when they
had their first experience.

A four-year period is usually too short for statistically
significant trends to emerge and there is no real evidence
from these figures that there is a trend to earlier experience for boys or girls. A recent American study of 4,240
teenage girls points to a 'dramatic change in teenage sexual
activity' in recent years: 'for those currently aged 19, 97%
were still virgins when they reached age 15, whereas only
91% of those now aged 15 reached the age in the virginal
state' (Kantner and Zelnik, 1972a, p.339). However, a
better comparison for our sample would be with Schofield's
figures. Unfortunately the only age breakdown given there
is for those under 15. In 1964 6% of 15-year-old boys and
2% of 15-year-old girls said that they were sexually experienced (Schofield, 1965, p.59). Comparing the 16-year-olds
in our sample who said they had had their first sexual
experience before they were 16, the proportions are 26% of
the boys and 12% of the girls. Some of this increase could
be accounted for by the difference in the age at which they
were asked the question, but it is unlikely that all of it
can be explained in this way, so some is probably due to an
actual increase.

One issue which immediately occurs is whether the age of
consent should be lowered. We do not know how many boys know
it is illegal to have intercourse with a girl under 16, or if
they do know, whether they are deterred by the knowledge.
Girls, although they themselves do not break the law by
having intercourse before they reach the age of consent, may
feel that what they are doing is disapproved of by people in
authority and so be afraid to seek birth control advice.
There is some feeling amongst those who specialise in offering contraceptive and counselling advice to the young, that
girls do not present themselves for help until they are 16,
even though they are having intercourse. There is one piece
of evidence suggesting this might be the case. A doctor who
has worked in teenage clinics said that girls came to the
clinic on their sixteenth birthday or soon after, when they
had in fact been having intercourse for some time (Hutchinson,
1976). In this sense the law which aims to protect could be
said to expose girls to the possibility of unplanned pregnancies. Our evidence suggests that one in eight girls is
likely to have sexual intercourse before the age of consent
and that this is a more common occurrence than it was ten

TABLE 6 Age of first experience by age and sex

Age of first sexual experience	MALES				FEMALES				ALL
	Age at time of interview				Age at time of interview				
	16	17	18	19	16	17	18	19	
	%	%	%	%	%	%	%	%	%
Before 16	26	32	32	33	13	13	14	10	22
16	5	16	17	24	9	17	12	16	15
17	-	2	12	12	-	9	21	19	10
18	-	-	4	4	-	-	5	14	3
19	-	-	-	1	-	-	-	8	1
Refused	5	2	4	3	3	5	5	6	4
No experience	64	48	31	23	75	56	43	27	45
Number = 100%	181	211	186	198	170	189	216	190	1,541

years ago. It would seem advisable therefore to consider a reduction in the age of consent if it would encourage girls to seek birth control advice from a reliable source.

Characteristics of those who said they were sexually experienced

It is difficult to begin to offer explanations for why some teenagers have sex before marriage and some do not. We know that in the past, in Western society at least, fear of pregnancy, fear of being found out (social stigma) and economic factors often prevented it. To a large extent these barriers no longer exist, and in some ways it is more appropriate now to ask why any teenagers wait until they are married. As Musgrove (1964, p.157) pointed out 12 years ago:

> The sexual powers and needs of adolescents need frank recognition; heterosexual experience in adolescence must be accepted, instruction in birth control given.... The contemporary social order and adult social attitudes are based, if not upon hypocrisy, on gigantic myths concerning the needs and nature of the young.

Religion

Most religions aim to act as a brake to physical expressions of desire or emotion before marriage, but people no longer seem to accept this. Except in the case of those who belonged to nonconformist churches, there was no difference in stated sexual experience between those who said they were not religious and those who said they were (54% were sexually experienced compared with 51% of those who identified themselves as belonging to a particular religion; but 40% of those who said they were Methodists or belonged to other nonconformist churches said they were sexually experienced).

Social class

Although Schofield reported no differences between social class groups and sexual experience, other studies have observed class differences. Kantner and Zelnik's findings (1972b) are complicated by racial mix but there was a correlation between socio-economic status and sexual experience in the 'expected' direction (i.e., more working-class teenagers said they had had sexual experience). Venner's study (1972) also suggested a relationship between higher levels of sexual experience and the lower socio-economic groups. At age 16, 7% of daughters of professional and managerial groups said they were experienced, compared with 21% of daughters of blue-collar

workers. Our findings are more in line with these more
recent American findings than with Schofield's. His data
suggest the same pattern although the differences were
not significant. The main class differences in our study
are between working-class boys and the rest. Analysis of
middle-class boys and girls and working-class girls showed
similar proportions saying they were sexually experienced
(49% of middle-class boys, 47% of middle-class girls, and
46% of working-class girls), whereas 60% of working-class
boys said they were sexually experienced. This finding
is not unexpected but seems important in beginning to
unravel the web of factors which account for early sexual
experience. Working-class boys are more likely to have
sexual intercourse because they are boys and society half
expects it; their parents are more likely to approve of
sex before marriage; they are more likely to be economically self-supporting and therefore to qualify for adult
status (see Reiss, 1970; Musgrove, 1964); and they have
nothing to fear in terms of becoming pregnant. Also peer
group influences are likely to encourage it, as Schofield
(1965) and Willmott (1966) pointed out. Middle-class boys
are subject to some of these influences, but in this study
they were more likely to be in full-time higher education
(28% compared with 8%) which means that they are not
usually economically independent and have 'more' to lose
if a girl they have sex with gets pregnant and they have
to support a family. Girls of both classes have the most
to lose (or gain) if they have sex and become pregnant.
The lack of social class differences between the girls is
surprising. Initially we had taken the traditional view
that working-class girls would be more attracted to early
marriage as a way out of dull jobs, and would therefore be
more likely to be sexually experienced. Is it possible
that the desire not to have children at an early age is
uniting women of all classes - or have working girls been
hitherto maligned?

USE OF BIRTH CONTROL

The preceding figures suggest that more young people are
having premarital sexual intercourse and some of them at
an early age. This may disturb some people and not
others. However, most people are likely to be concerned
with whether the young people protect themselves from the
risk of unwanted pregnancies. The figures from this survey
suggest that to some extent they do. Of the 790 who said
they were sexually experienced, only 66 (8%) said that
they had never used any method of birth control. They were

asked three questions about the methods they had used:
'Have you ever used any method of birth control when you
have had sexual intercourse?' '...which was the first
method you used?' 'Can you say what method you used most
recently?' The types of methods they had used show a
progression from the less reliable methods which they used
at first to the more reliable methods they had used most
recently. Whereas 27% mentioned withdrawal and the 'safe'
period as the first method they had used, only 14% claimed
those as the most recent methods to be used. Similarly,
52% mentioned using the sheath as their first method of
contraception, and this fell to 37% who named it as the
most recent method used. In comparison, the proportion
who mentioned the pill as the first method of contraception used was 11%, compared with 39% who said it was
the most recent method used.

The sheath was the method most commonly used by these
teenagers and had been used on at least one occasion by
74% of the sexually experienced. The pill was the second
most frequent method and had been used by 48%. Withdrawal
came third in this league table, with 40% mentioning it
as a method they had used. This is not a particularly
useful guide to contraceptive behaviour since the figures
include male and female users. When the methods are
broken down by sex the pattern is slightly different.
For the girls in the sample, use of the sheath was
mentioned by 71% of those with sexual experience; the pill
came second and had been used by 59%; withdrawal was the
third most commonly used method with 35% mentioning it as
a method they had used. For boys there was a reversal of
the pill and withdrawal. For them the proportions are:
sheath 76%, withdrawal 45%, and the pill 39%.

Tables 7 and 8 show the proportions of boys and girls
who said they had ever used these methods, the first
method they used, and the method they had used most
recently. Of the girls who had ever used the pill, 10%
(22) had stopped taking it - or had not used it as the
most recent method. Ten of them had changed to the
sheath; four had used withdrawal and three had used
chemicals as their most recent methods; one girl had been
fitted with a coil. For seven of the girls these changes
can be explained by the fact that they had got married
and perhaps felt they did not need to use such a reliable
method. Four other girls were not currently having a
sexual relationship and possibly felt the pill was un-
suitable - but half of the girls (11) were having sexual
relationships and the most likely reason they stopped
taking the pill is that they did not like this method or
the services through which they obtained it. Unfortunately,

we did not ask why methods had been changed, so this is
speculation.

TABLE 7   Proportions of sexually experienced 16-19-year-
olds who had ever used particular methods of birth control

Method	Male	Female	All sexually experienced
	%	%	%
Sheath	76	71	74
Withdrawal	45	35	40
Pill	39	59	48
Safe period	14	8	12
Chemicals	4	6	5
Cap	2	1	1
I.U.D.	2	1	1
Other	-	2	1
No methods ever used	10	6	8
Number (= 100%)*	433	357	790
Average number of different methods of birth control used	1.8	1.8	1.8

* Percentages add to more than 100 as some had used more
  than one method.

   Of the girls who had ever used the sheath, over half
(51%) had changed to the pill and 40% were still using
the sheath.   The others had changed to withdrawal (6%)
and chemicals and safe period (3%).   For those girls who
said they had used withdrawal (126), a quarter (26%) were
still using it and nearly half (48%) had changed to the
pill.   A fifth (21%) had used the sheath as the most
recent method and 5% had used the safe period and chemicals.
   The majority of girls do seem to progress to using more
reliable methods, but a small proportion change to less
reliable methods.   Their reasons for doing so are probably
related to preference or partner preference, or reluctance
to use birth control services to get more reliable methods.

Age and types of methods used

Analysis of the methods used indicates that both sexes move
on to using the more reliable methods, whatever their age.
The proportion of 16-year-old boys using withdrawal as the

TABLE 8 First method and most recent methods of birth control used by sexually experienced 16-19-year-olds

Method	Males			Females			Both sexes		
	At first sexual experience	First method	Most recent method	At first sexual experience	First method	Most recent method	At first sexual experience	First method	Most recent method
	%	%	%	%	%	%	%	%	%
Sheath	37	54	44	36	51	28	37	52	37
Withdrawal	9	27	13	10	23	10	10	25	12
Pill	4	6	28	8	17	53	6	11	39
Safe period	2	3	2	1	2	2	1	2	2
Chemicals	1	1	1	1	2	1	1	1	1
Cap	–	–	–	–	–	–	–	–	–
I.U.D.	–	–	1	–	–	–	–	–	–
Others	–	1	1	1	3	2	–	2	1
No method	47	10	10	43	6	6	45	8	8
Number of sexually experienced (= 100%)*	433			357			790		

* Percentages add to more than 100 because some had used more than one method (e.g. sheath with chemicals).

first method dropped from 37% to 24% when they were asked
about the method they had used most recently. Table 9
shows that the pattern is the same for 19-year-old boys
and also for the girls. The major shift for the younger
boys is from withdrawal to the sheath and for the older
boys from withdrawal and the sheath to the pill. The
girls tend to move on to the pill.

TABLE 9   First and most recent methods of birth control
used by age and sex

Methods	Males			
	16-year-olds		19-year-olds	
	First	Most recent	First	Most recent
	%	%	%	%
Withdrawal	37	24	34	14
Sheath	57	65	57	34
Pill	2	6	7	52
Others	4	5	2	–
Number using birth control (= 100%)	49	49	137	137
% of sexually experienced young people who had never used any method	11%		6%	

	Females			
Withdrawal	30	15	23	8
Sheath	61	45	53	22
Pill	6	36	19	67
Others	3	4	5	3
Number using birth control (= 100%)	33	33	120	120
% of sexually experienced young people who had never used any method	11%		4%	

Although these figures give a fairly favourable picture
of sexually active teenagers taking action to avoid
pregnancy, it is necessary to consider the risks they take
if they use the less reliable methods or if they use birth

control haphazardly. We know that 8% of them never used any methods, that 4% only used withdrawal, and a further 1% used the safe period and chemicals. This means that a total of 15% of boys and 11% of the girls used no methods or had used methods with a high chance of failure.

A second important consideration is the stage at which they begin to use contraception. Just over half (54%) of the sexually experienced teenagers said that they had used some method of birth control on the first occasion they had intercourse, and just over a third (36%) claimed that they had always used a method. But of the ones who had used a method on the first occasion, 22% had used either withdrawal, the safe period or chemicals. In addition, of those who had used birth control on the first occasion, a third (33%) admitted that afterwards they had sometimes taken a chance. Altogether half (55%) of the sexually experienced admitted that they did not always use birth control, and of those who had always used it, 8% used the less reliable methods (withdrawal, the safe period and chemicals).

There are differences in the methods used by those who had used contraception on the first occasion and continued to use birth control regularly, those who used a method on the first occasion but then subsequently took a chance, and those who had not used a method on the first occasion. Table 10 shows that both boys and girls who had always used birth control were more likely to start off with the sheath than those who started using birth control after their first experience. They in turn were more likely to use withdrawal as their first method. This would seem to confirm that those who used contraception on the first occasion and continued to do so also used a more reliable method to help them avoid pregnancy.

An analysis by age of these three types of birth control users suggests that some impression may have been made by campaigns to encourage use of birth control. The younger boys were more likely to say that they had always used birth control than the older ones (42% of 16-year-old boys said this compared with 25% of the 19-year-olds). The fact that a third of all these boys used withdrawal as the first method is not as encouraging as it might be, and indicates room for improvement, but is better than their not using any method at all. There were no differences in the first method used by the younger and older girls within the three types of users. The younger boys and girls have, of course, not had as much time to take chances as the older ones, but the fact that the 16-year-old boys were no less likely to have used a method on the first occasion, and that two-thirds of them had used the sheath, is a

TABLE 10 First method of contraceptive used and the stage at which it was used

1st method used	MALES			FEMALES		
	Method used on 1st occasion and always thereafter	Method used on 1st occasion but later took a chance	No method used on 1st occasion but afterwards	Method used on 1st occasion and always thereafter	Method used on 1st occasion but later took a chance	No method used on 1st occasion but afterwards
	%	%	%	%	%	%
Sheath	72	69	46	66	65	38
Withdrawal	14	26	47	15	25	35
Pill	10	4	6	16	7	25
Others	4	1	1	3	3	2
Number using birth control (= 100%)	139	85	158	140	55	130

hopeful sign. There were no class differences in the
methods the young people had chosen to use on the first
occasion.

However, although the picture given by these teenagers
is of fairly widespread use of contraception, at least
half of them are exposing themselves or their partners to
the risk of pregnancy at some point in their sexual
careers.

Effective use of birth control

Since it is no longer realistic (or even desirable) to
look at the characteristics of those who do not wait until
they are married to have sex, we should try to look at
what makes young people control their fertility effectively.

One way to do it is to look at those people who have
failed to control it - those girls who had had abortions,
those who said they had married because they were pregnant
and those single girls who had children. This approach,
however, rests on the assumption that these girls did not
want to become pregnant - and since we did not ask this
question it would be wrong to proceed on the assumption
that they did not. It seems more appropriate therefore
to look at the characteristics of those sexually experienced young people who had always used birth control
methods (since this is a sign that they are serious about
fertility control) and compare them with those who said
they had never used any methods of birth control.

Although there were only 66 sexually experienced young
people who said they had never used any method of birth
control, the majority of them were working-class boys
(68%). Two per cent of middle-class, sexually experienced,
young people had never used any method of birth control
compared with 12% of the working-class group. Over half
of them (58%) were from the younger age groups; 14% of
the 16 and 17-year-olds had not used birth control compared
with 6% of the 18 and 19-year-olds. It looks as if those
who do not attempt to control their fertility are the
younger working-class boys, who are not as likely to be
involved in stable relationships. In comparison those
who said they had always used birth control were more
likely to be middle-class girls from the older age groups.
Fifty-three per cent of sexually experienced middle-class
girls had always used birth control compared with 32% of
sexually experienced working-class girls; 43% of sexually
experienced middle-class boys had always used birth control
compared with 25% of sexually experienced working-class
boys. There were no class differences in the type of birth
control first used.

SUMMARY

Young people's attitudes to sex before marriage are in
line with what has been described as the 'widespread'
view in this country - approval in the context of a
stable relationship and if care is taken to avoid unwanted
pregnancy.

Compared with Schofield's figures of ten years ago,
there seems to have been an increase in the proportion of
16-19-year-old boys and girls saying they are sexually
experienced. There is a possibility that some of this
increase is due to the fact that young people feel that
it is more acceptable to say that they are sexually
experienced now than they did ten years ago. There also
seems to be a trend to earlier sexual experience.
Working-class boys are more likely to say they are
sexually experienced than other groups. There is scope
for consideration of changes in the law on the age of
consent, if it would encourage younger girls to use birth
control.

In the main the sexually active young people had used
methods of birth control, but only a third reported that
they had done so on every occasion. A small proportion
said they had never used any methods (8%), and two out of
every three of these were boys.

3

KNOWLEDGE OF BIRTH CONTROL AND VENEREAL DISEASE AND ATTITUDES TO ABORTION

Attempting to 'test' knowledge in an interview is a
difficult task. To begin with the person being interviewed almost always knows that he or she is being tested
and often resents it. Second, the assumption that an
individual's knowledge can be tested is a dubious one.
It may be that all that can be done is to measure an
individual's capacity to produce answers in a particular
setting. Because of these problems, three different ways
of asking for birth control knowledge were used in this
study: open-ended questions, questions about the advantages, disadvantages and reliability of each method, and
finally a set of self-administered questions for completion
after the interview. (These questions are attached as
Appendix IV.) Table 11 shows the methods of birth control
mentioned spontaneously ('Could you tell me what contraceptives or birth control methods there are for people to
use, if they don't want to have a baby?') by boys and
girls, side by side with the proportions who said they had
heard of individual methods when they were checked off by
the interviewer. (The interviewer said, 'I'm going to
read out this list that I've got of various possible
methods of preventing pregnancy. Could you say if you've
heard of _____? Could you tell me what you think is the
main advantage of _____? Could you tell me what you think
is the main disadvantage of _____? Would you describe_____
as a very reliable method, fairly reliable, not very
reliable?' Each method was mentioned in turn.)

TABLE 11   Methods of birth control mentioned by sex

Methods	Methods mentioned spontaneously		Methods ever heard of	
	Male	Female	Male	Female
	%	%	%	%
Pill	86	95	99	99
Cap	29	35	65	80
Coil	43	66	65	90
Sheath	87	79	98	96
Chemicals	25	31	47	57
Withdrawal	20	16	81	84
Rhythm/safe period	14	17	66	77
Male Sterilisation	28	20	94	96
Female Sterilisation			91	96
Abortion	5	1	-	-
Could not name any methods	3	2	-	-
Number asked (= 100%)	782	774	782	774

The pill and the sheath were mentioned most often by both boys and girls at each question. The fact that more boys mentioned the sheath spontaneously is probably because it is the method they are most likely to use and are responsible for using. It is also possibly the one method they are told about more often than girls. Surprisingly, perhaps, the coil was the method mentioned third most frequently at the spontaneous question by both boys and girls. The proportions spontaneously mentioning withdrawal and the safe period were low but increased substantially when they were asked to say if they had heard of these methods - an indication either that young people do not think of these two methods as methods of birth control, or that they are reluctant to mention them.

Hearing about birth control and 'knowing' about it are two different things, so asking the young people to mention the main advantage and the main disadvantage of each method was one way of beginning to understand in more detail how deep their knowledge of birth control was.

The pill

Over half the girls (52%) and a third (36%) of the boys
said that the main advantage of the pill was its
reliability. Another quarter of the girls (26%) and boys
(27%) said convenience and ease of use was the main
advantage:
    'It's about the easiest, really. It's simple, no
    bother.'
The main disadvantages were seen as specific side effects
(such as thrombosis, high blood pressure and weight gain)
by 42% of the boys and 56% of the girls:
    'It's supposed to make you go all big around the hips.'
Some of the comments revealed uncertainty, if not wrong
information:
    'Some say it can make you sterile, don't they?'
    'I don't know. Does anybody know? I suppose there are
    side effects.'
    'I should think you need a rest from it every so often.'
A further 4% of boys and 3% of girls said it was not safe
or 'healthy' to take it without specific mention of side
effects. In addition, 14% of the sample (19% of boys and
10% of girls) said that they did not know of or could not
name any disadvantages. Some of the young people named
the problem of remembering to take it every day as a
disadvantage (13% of boys and 16% of girls). Some
mentioned long-term disadvantages such as it being the
cause of cancer and sterility (8% of boys and 8% of girls)
and a few (5% of boys and 4% of girls) named a mixture of
other disadvantages, like the problem of having to go to
the doctor or clinic for it. A small group of boys (9%)
and girls (5%) said that there were no disadvantages of
taking the pill. In terms of reliability, the pill was
generally seen as the most reliable method except for
sterilisation. Table 12 shows that nearly two-thirds of
the young people said it was very reliable compared with
less than a fifth who said the sheath was very reliable.
Even so, a third regarded it as less than very reliable.
The differences between those who said it was a very
reliable method and those who thought it was fairly
reliable or not very reliable followed the expected
pattern. More girls than boys said the pill was very
reliable (66% compared with 55%) and so did more of those
who were sexually experienced (62% compared with 47%).
Middle-class boys and girls were more likely than working-
class teenagers to say the pill was very reliable. Among
those from working-class families, the older teenagers
were more likely to say that this method was very reliable
(62% compared with 43% of the younger ones). There were

TABLE 12 Reliability of different methods of birth control

	Pill	Sheath	With- drawal	Safe period	Chemi- cals	Cap	I.U.D.	Male	Female sterilisation
	%	%	%	%	%	%	%	%	%
Very reliable	61	18	2	4	4	8	19	87	85
Fairly reliable	30	51	9	22	29	46	40	8	9
Not very reliable	3	24	85	62	40	14	11	1	1
Don't know	6	7	4	12	27	32	30	4	5
Number who had heard of each method, excluding inadequate answers (= 100%)	1,533	1,491	1,268	1,099	794	1,107	1,187	1,447	1,419

no differences with regard to views about pill reliability
between those who had named different people as being the
most helpful for learning about birth control.

The sheath

As shown in Chapter 2, the sheath was the method most
commonly used by sexually experienced young people. Its
main advantages were seen by the boys as reliability (25%)
and the fact that it was easy to get and cheap (24%).
Another one in five boys (20%) mentioned the fact that it
was handy for 'spur of the moment' occasions and easy to
use, but 13% said they did not know of any advantages and
7% said there were no advantages. Other advantages
mentioned were that it offered some protection from
venereal diseases (4%) and that there were no side effects
(2%). The girls had a rather different view of the sheath.
More of them said there were not any advantages or could
not say what they might be (14% and 27% respectively).
The advantage mentioned most frequently by the girls was
the handy and easy to use one (16%), followed by easy to
get and cheap (14%), and reliability (12%). Some girls
(7%) mentioned the fact that it was a method boys took
the responsibility for:
    'It's a protection a man can take instead of a woman
    having to take it all the time.'
The rest gave a variety of advantages, including avoiding
venereal diseases (2%) and the fact that there were no
side effects (4%).
    Boys and girls had different priorities too in mention-
ing the main disadvantage of the sheath. For the boys the
most common one was the fact that it was unreliable and
could split or come off (38%):
    'In so many ways it's pretty vile - the discomfort and
    the fact that it could have a hole in it.'
Nearly one in five (18%) said they could not think of any
disadvantages, and 12% said there were not any. But 16%
said that it was uncomfortable and 'spoiled sex':
    'It's not like the real thing. It's a bit like washing
    your feet with your socks on.'
Others mentioned the fact that it was difficult to use
(9%):
    'Well it could be difficult to keep it up.'
Four per cent said that it was a nuisance to remember:
    'It could be awkward if you haven't got one on you at
    the time.'
    The girls were more likely to say they did not know
about disadvantages (29%) but less likely to say there

were not any (2%). Nearly half of them (45%) mentioned
the fact that it was unreliable, and one in ten mentioned
discomfort or the fact that it spoiled sex (10%). The
rest mentioned difficulty or awkwardness in using the
sheath (7%), and the fact that it was a nuisance to
remember (2%).

In terms of reliability, half the young people who
answered the question said it was fairly reliable (51%),
a quarter said it was not very reliable (24%), and 18%
said it was very reliable. Boys were more likely than
girls to say it was a very reliable method (28% compared
with 8%). Overall it was considered the most reliable of
the non-medical methods.

Withdrawal

This was the third most commonly used method, and 85% of
the young people considered it was not a very reliable
method. There were no differences between the advantages
mentioned by boys and girls, and it seems sensible that
about half the young people should say there were not any
advantages (46%). Another 16% did not know or could not
mention any advantages. Of those who did mention an
advantage, the one mentioned most frequently was the fact
that it was not necessary to bother with devices or
'preliminaries' (13%). After this, small numbers mentioned
the fact that it was free (5%), that it was fairly reliable
(5%), that it was quite pleasant to use (4%), and that it
was better than nothing (3%).

The disadvantages were spelled out more vigorously and
there were differences between the boys and girls. Over
half the girls mentioned its unreliability (52%, compared
with 42% of the boys), and 28% of the boys mentioned the
difficulties of using self-control to withdraw at the
right time:
        'It depends on human decision in the middle of making
        love. It's difficult to be precise.'
        'You've got to be quick - may get over-excited.'
This was mentioned by 16% of the girls. Another 16% of
the boys and 13% of the girls said it was not a 'natural'
thing to do and could be frustrating:
        'It's frustrating for the man; well I suppose for the
        woman as well.'
One in ten (10% of the boys and 13% of the girls) said
that they did not know of any disadvantages. Those who
were sexually experienced were more likely to say it was
not a very reliable method.

On the whole, and apart from those who said they had

not heard of the different methods, the young people seemed
well aware of the relative merits of the three methods
they are apparently most likely to use. This is not quite
the same thing as having a 'satisfactory' working knowledge,
and so we look next at their answers to the self-administered questions.

Before the findings are discussed, there are a number
of reservations about these kind of data which should be
mentioned. There is the chance element, always present
in multi-choice questions where some people who do not
know, 'guess' the answer correctly. There is also the
possibility of the wording of the questions being mis-
understood. In addition, not all of the alternatives are
right or wrong, but this has been covered where possible
by classifying as wrong only the answers which, if
practised, could lead to pregnancy.

There were no differences between the number of right
answers given by all the boys and girls, but there were
differences between those who were sexually experienced
and those who were not. The highest mean scores on the
self-administered questions were achieved by girls and
boys who said they were sexually experienced (4.5 and 4.3
correct answers). Girls and boys who said they were not
sexually experienced had mean scores of 3.3 and 3.6
respectively. The difference between those who were
sexually experienced and those who were not sexually
experienced was only to be expected, since the former
were more likely to have experience of using the methods.
A closer look at individual questions and analysis of
those who said they had used the methods gives a clearer
picture of the proportions using methods in ignorance.
Table 13 shows what proportion of those who said they had
ever used a method got the answer 'right', compared with
those who had never used it and those who were not sexually
experienced.

The table shows, reassuringly perhaps, that those who
had used the methods were more likely to give the right
answers than those who had not (with the exception of male
answers on withdrawal). Also, girls were more likely to
give correct answers to the questions on the pill, chemicals and the safe period, less likely to give the correct
answer to the sheath question, and had less trust in withdrawal. Although the proportions of both boys and girls
giving correct answers to the questions about the safe
period are low, relatively small numbers of young people
used this method. The figures for withdrawal are less
worrying since we know that the majority of young people
considered it a very unreliable method anyway. Also, those
young people who answered 'false' to this question may have

TABLE 13   Proportions who gave correct answers about using methods of birth control by sex and users

Methods	Those who said they had used methods		Those who had not used methods (including those who said they were not sexually experienced)	
	Male	Female	Male	Female
Questions on self-administered questionnaire (see Appendix IV)				
Sheath (Q.1a)	85% (330)	85% (253)	69% (452)	55% (521)
Pill (Q.2a)	80% (168)	86% (210)	62% (614)	67% (564)
Withdrawal (Q.3)	72% (193)	67% (126)	67% (589)	50% (648)
Safe period (Q.4)	55% (62)	59% (29)	26% (720)	41% (745)
Chemicals (Q.6)	* 61% (18)	100% (20)	25% (764)	36% (754)

* Based on less than 20.
( )Numbers in brackets are base number.

considered withdrawal totally unreliable, but had used it
before they acquired that view. However, there are
obviously a number of young people who use methods of
contraception about which they are not fully informed.
Amongst the users there were no age or class differences
between the young people who got the answers right and
those who did not, except on the question of using the
sheath, where working-class boys were less likely to get
the answer right (82% of these boys gave the correct
answer compared with 90% of middle-class boys). If we
look at all the young people and all the methods, middle-
class boys and girls were more likely to achieve a higher
score than young people from working-class families.
Table 14 shows the proportions of each giving correct
answers and their mean score.

TABLE 14   Social class and sex differences in the number
of correct answers given to questions on the use of birth
control methods

Number of 'right' answers	Middle class		Working class	
	Male	Female	Male	Female
	%	%	%	%
0	2	4	3	3
1	3	5	7	10
2	7	10	14	14
3	20	18	19	19
4	26	17	23	18
5	19	19	19	18
6	13	13	10	11
7	8	10	4	6
8	2	4	1	1
9	–	–	–	–
Number = 100%	310	289	431	427
Mean score =	4.3	4.2	3.8	3.7

The evidence suggests that not only were working-class
boys less likely to use methods of birth control (see
Chapter 2) and more likely to be sexually experienced, but
they were also less likely to give as many correct
answers. Table 15 shows the mean scores of middle-class
and working-class boys and the most recent methods used;
in all the categories of method users, working-class boys
had a lower score, although the numbers of pill and withdrawal users were too small for the differences to be
significant.

TABLE 15 Mean scores on birth control knowledge of
sexually experienced boys by social class and methods used

Most recent method used	Middle-class males	Working-class males
	Mean score	Mean score
Pill users	5.0 (46)	4.5 (71)
Sheath users	4.5 (78)	4.0 (102)
Withdrawal users	4.1 (18)	4.0 (39)
No methods used	6.3 (3)	3.2 (39)
All (middle- and working-class) sexually experienced boys	4.7 (152)	4.0 (258)

( ) Numbers of boys involved in each mean are given in
    brackets after mean.

Over half the boys (55%) and girls (58%) said they
would like to know more about birth control. Of those
who were sexually experienced, over half (55% of the boys
and 50% of the girls) said they would like to know more
about birth control. The methods they specifically wanted
to know more about were the coil (75%), chemicals (74%),
the cap (72%), the pill (71%), the 'safe' period (62%),
sterilisation (61%), withdrawal (54%) and the sheath
(53%). Those who said they knew enough about birth control
did, for the most part, achieve higher scores than those
who said they would like to know more, but there were no
differences between the scores of the 16-year-old boys and
girls who said they wanted to know more and who knew
enough.

TABLE 16 Mean scores of those who knew enough about birth
control and those who wanted to know more by sex and age

	Males		Females	
Age	Knew enough about birth control	Wanted to know more about birth control	Knew enough about birth control	Wanted to know more about birth control
16	3.8 (74)	3.5 (107)	4.1 (58)	3.6 (109)
17	4.3 (93)	3.6 (119)	4.1 (70)	3.3 (117)
18	4.4 (90)	3.9 (95)	4.6 (83)	3.9 (133)
19	4.7 (97)	4.0 (104)	4.7 (103)	3.8 (88)
All young people	4.3 (354)	3.7 (425)	4.4 (314)	3.6 (447)

( ) Numbers in brackets are base numbers for means.

These findings suggest that teenagers become more knowledgeable about birth control after they have sexual experience and once they have used particular methods. This is reassuring in one sense, but if it means that knowledge is gained through trial and error, then more preparation at an earlier stage is necessary to avoid attendant risks. A group of young people who can be identified as less well informed than others are the working-class boys. Since they are also more likely to be sexually experienced, there would seem to be a clear case for encouraging their greater responsibility for contraceptive use through better and more accessible birth control education. The following section discusses the girls who had had abortions - but they were not solely responsible for their unwanted pregnancies. It is possible that if more attention were paid to informing boys about risks of pregnancy and the difficulties young girls face if they do have or want an abortion, they would be more likely to share in contraceptive discussions and use.

EXPERIENCES OF PREGNANCY AND ABORTION

In this study, 18 of the 774 girls (that is, 2%) said that they had had an abortion. Using published data for 1971, 1972, 1973 and 1974, we calculated that we should have had 34 cases. It is easy to understand that this is an area in which untruthful answers might be given, but it may also be speculated that the under-representation may have occurred because these girls were more likely to refuse to be interviewed. Even if the sample had not been under-represented, we would only be dealing with 4.4% of the age group. In the light of the publicity given to this question, it seems sensible to point out that 95.6% of the girls in the age group will not have had an abortion.

Most of the girls (11) said they had had their abortions when they were 16, only one girl was younger than that and she said she was 14. The small numbers mean that cross-analysis is not particularly useful and there are no basic characteristics which mark the girls out as being different. One interesting fact which may be a pointer is that over half of them (10) had never had birth control lessons in school, and seven of them, even after their experience of abortion, said they felt they needed to know more about birth control methods. The birth control history of these girls is not markedly different from the rest of the sexually experienced girls in the study, and certainly does not indicate that they were particularly careless.

Three of the girls (17%) said they had used birth control
on the first occasion they had sex and had always used it
after that. One had used withdrawal, the other two the
sheath. These girls seem to be the unlucky ones. One had
become a pill user since the abortion, and the other two
were not having a sexual relationship. A third of the
girls (6) had not used birth control on the first occasion
they had sex, but said that afterwards they had used birth
control more often than they had taken a chance. They too
had used the sheath (4) and withdrawal (2) as the first
method of birth control. More unlucky ones! Two-fifths
of the girls (7) had not used birth control on the first
occasion and admitted that they had taken a chance more
often than they had used birth control. Again when they
had used methods they mentioned the sheath and withdrawal.
Three of them were currently using the pill. One girl
said she had used birth control on the first occasion but
had then taken a chance more often than she had used birth
control, and withdrawal was the only method she had used.
Only one girl said she had never used any birth control
methods, and she was a Roman Catholic.

Not all unmarried girls who become pregnant choose to
have an abortion, and 6% of the girls in this study had
children. The majority of them were married (72%), but
nearly two-thirds of these girls (64%) said they had
married because they were pregnant. Three of those who
had married (9%) had afterwards separated from their
husbands. Altogether, of the 64 girls who said they had
had pregnancies, 28% had 'chosen' abortion, 33% had
'chosen' marriage, and 20% had 'chosen' illegitimacy.
The remaining 19% had married first and then become
pregnant.

Again the numbers are small for useful analysis,
but if we look only at the single girls who had had
children and those married girls who said they married
because they were pregnant (34 altogether) we see that
pregnancy seems to have been at least partly due to inadequate knowledge of birth control. Although it may be
due to hindsight, over half of them said that they felt
they had learned about birth control too late, and three
of these said they had never learned about it. A high
proportion (72%) said they had not used any method of
birth control on the first occasion they had sex, and
since then the methods they had used tended to be the less
reliable methods. On the first occasion they had used
contraceptives, a third (32%) said they had used the
sheath, another third (32%) had used withdrawal, 9% had
never used any methods, and 7% had used the 'safe' period
or chemicals on their own. Even after pregnancy, nearly

half of these girls (42%) said they felt they would like
to know more about birth control methods.

On the whole, although the figures are small, it looks
as though the girls who became pregnant (except for the
girls who married first) were trying to control their
fertility. They chose to use the less reliable methods,
the non-medical methods, and some of them felt that they
did not know enough about birth control. The fact that
three-fifths of abortions (61%) were carried out at the
age of 16 is an indication that these girls were having
sex before the age of consent and therefore might not have
felt able to approach a doctor for advice.

ATTITUDES TO ABORTION

The majority of young people expressed strong feelings
about abortion and, contrary to what might have been
expected, a greater proportion disapproved than approved.
When they were asked to say whether they approved, disapproved or had mixed feelings about abortion, 38% said
that on the whole they approved, 49% disapproved, and the
remaining 13% had mixed feelings which were equally
balanced for and against. Most young people expressed
strong views about abortion. When asked, 'What do you
think of abortion?', over a third (36%) made comments
which could be classified as strong disapproval, half of
them mentioning the word 'murder' or 'killing':
  'It should be avoided at all costs - I don't believe
  in killing unborn children.'
  'I don't like it - it's just like shooting a calf.'
Others felt it was wrong except in specific circumstances:
11% mentioned rape or medical reasons as a justification:
  'You've got to have it. But my own personal view is
  that I don't like it - although I feel it's necessary
  in certain circumstances like rape or mental instabil-
  ity.'
Some (13%) said it was preferable to producing unwanted
children:
  'It's killing human life - but if it's that or misery
  for the baby and yourself then it's better - if you
  know you're going to bring a baby into the world and
  can't keep it.'
A small group (3%) mentioned that it should be allowed
only if the mother was very young and another 5% felt that
people should be responsible for their own actions:
  'I think it's wrong - it's her own fault for getting
  into trouble. They should think of these things.'

Over half of those who approved of abortion explained
their views mostly in terms of avoiding human misery:
> 'It's a good thing. Having a baby can lead to a great
> deal of unhappiness for a girl or boy - him if he's
> forced to marry her, and the child when it grows up.'

A further 23% made comments which revealed a mixture of
feelings:
> 'I don't really agree with it but it's an easy way out
> for the mother - too easy sometimes. I think I'd say
> I was mixed really, I can't make my mind up.'

Finally, a small group (5%) avoided making moral judgments,
saying that it was neither right nor wrong, but necessary:
> 'It's a positive method of solving a problem if you can
> afford it.'

Girls, for whom abortion is a more directly practical
problem, were less likely to say they approved than boys.
Table 17 shows the differences between them and the class
differences.

TABLE 17   Attitudes to abortion by social class and sex

Attitudes	Females		Males		All
	Middle class	Working class	Middle class	Working class	
	%	%	%	%	%
Approve	22	11	34	25	22
Mixed - more to approve	11	7	11	11	16
Mixed - equally balanced	18	18	15	11	13
Mixed - more to disapprove	18	14	10	11	9
Disapprove	31	50	30	42	40
Number = 100%	286*	425*	308*	422*	1,540**

* These figures exclude 16 young people whose answers
  were inadequate.
** Including 99 young people whose fathers' occupations
  were not classified as either middle class or working
  class, but excluding inadequate answers.

These findings have implications for the proposed
changes in the abortion law. Girls from working-class
families are more likely to disapprove of abortion, and
yet are more likely to be exposed to the need for one,
since the data show that they are more likely to have

unprotected intercourse. (Only 32% of all sexually
experienced working-class girls said that they always used
a method of birth control compared with 53% of all sexually
experienced middle-class girls.) If they do become pregnant they are likely to experience greater emotional conflict than if they approved of abortion, which in itself
could lead to delay in seeking help and advice. In
research for the Lane Committee, Cartwright and Lucas
(1974) established that single women having an abortion
tended to consult for pregnancy confirmation at a later
stage than married women.

The girls were asked a more specific question to find
out, in personal terms, in which circumstances they might
consider having an abortion, and 29% said that they would
never consider it in any circumstances. Another 29% said
they would consider it only if there were strong medical
reasons:

'If the doctor says there is something going to be
really wrong with the baby I would have an abortion,
otherwise I would have the baby.'
'If it was going to endanger my life or the baby
wasn't going to be normal.'

These were typical comments. Altogether over half (58%)
of the girls could not see themselves having abortions
unless there was a risk to life or health. Over a third
(36%) described what might be called social reasons for
considering an abortion:

'If I was pregnant by mistake and the father I realised
would be no good; if the money situation was desperate
and the child would be worse off in the end, and if
I'd have to give it up to adopt.'

Within this group financial support was mentioned as a
consideration by 9%, the baby being unwanted by the girl
or the father or her parents by 7%, and no family support
and not wanting to marry the father by 21%.

Finally, 11% said they would think seriously about
abortion if it looked as if their future would be ruined,
and 7% felt uncertain what they would do. (Percentages
here do not add to 100% because some gave more than one
circumstance; but the 58% and 36% are exclusive.)

Since the attitude of the father often plays a part in
a girl's reactions towards pregnancy, the boys were asked
in what circumstances they would encourage a girlfriend
to have an abortion. Nearly a third (31%) said they never
would because they were against or disapproved of abortion.
A further 10% said they would only if there was a medical
risk or health hazard:

'Well, it depends; if they think the child's going to
have brain damage and you wouldn't like to see it
walking on the streets....'

So altogether 41% of the boys could not see themselves
encouraging abortion if they were involved, except for
medical reasons. One in seven of the boys (16%) opted
out of the question by saying they would leave it to the
girl to decide:
    'I don't think it's really my line or for me to say.
    It's up to the girl whether to have one.'
But the remaining 43% described a variety of situations,
some of which were social, others more personal considerations. One in five (21%) said they would encourage it if
they did not want to marry the girl, if it was too soon
to settle down or the girl did not want to marry them:
    'If I didn't fancy settling down with her.'
    'If we weren't really thinking of getting married.'
Eight per cent said the fact that marriage was impossible
for financial reasons or because they were too young would
be a consideration, and another 5% mentioned family disapproval of the marriage or their refusal to support the
girl. Others (6%) mentioned the girl's age as a circumstance in which they might consider encouraging her to
have an abortion:
    'If she was younger than 16 I would.'
    The fact that over half the girls and over 40% of the
boys expressed disapproval (and often horror) of abortion
is an indication that young people are not encouraged to
have sex because abortion is more easily available now.
The evidence on contraceptive use presented in Chapter 2
suggests that the majority of girls and boys use birth
control methods, and girls certainly do not regard
abortion as an alternative to contraception. Efforts
might be better directed at changing male attitudes to
contraception and encouraging responsibility in relationships, than trying to change the law so that a few girls
may be 'punished' for their inability to say 'no' or
'only if'.

KNOWLEDGE OF VENEREAL DISEASE

Almost all the young people in this study had heard of
VD (98%), and the majority (88%) knew more or less how it
was transmitted. Within this group there were three
types of answers (they were asked, 'Could you tell me how
you catch VD?'): 40% said through sexual intercourse
without mentioning the fact that it was necessary for one
of the partners to be infected:
    'Through intercourse. (PROBE) No, it's a load of
    bollocks that you can get it off toilet seats.'

But 31% did give the 'right' answer, specifically mentioning that it was caught by having intercourse with someone
who had it:
    'Sexual intercourse from someone who's already
    infected.'
    'It's a germ picked up through having sexual inter-
    course with someone who's got it.'
Another 20% said it was caught from dirty people, by being
promiscuous, or by sleeping with someone who had been
promiscuous:
    'Going around with everybody, people, layabouts who
    hang around beaches and alleyways, who sleep outside,
    you know, dirty people, sort of thing.'
    'They said that it was if you met a boy and if he kept
    going from one girl to another and then had intercourse
    with you, he might know about it and wouldn't care and
    you would end up with it as well.'
Not everyone thought the lavatory seat was a 'load of
bollocks', because 6% gave this as the way to catch VD,
and another 3% thought 'kissing' could be the cause. A
further 6% said they did not know or could not say how it
was transmitted.
    Although these teenagers knew what VD was, and most of
them knew how it was transmitted, only 17% mentioned that
use of the sheath helped to avoid catching it. Over a
third (37%) did not know a way to avoid it, and the rest
emphasised 'keeping clean' and not being promiscuous:
    'Choose the right partner - I wouldn't go out with a
    dirty girl - you can usually tell the type of girl
    who's probably got it. These hippie girls and that.
    The only time I've ever risked it is down _____
    where they're easy. When my mate and I go down there
    we take a bottle of Dettol and cotton wool when we go -
    better take precautions. My girl and I, we have a
    bath afterwards, and sometimes before if we can.'
    'Don't have it off with scrubbers.'
A more pessimistic view:
    'There aren't any [ways to avoid it]. If you have
    sex with anybody else and they've got it, that's it.'
    When they were asked to describe the symptoms which
might make them think they had VD, there was a lot more
uncertainty. Part of it was probably due to embarrassment
and not wanting to name genitalia - but mostly it seemed
due to lack of precise knowledge. What seems to happen
is that VD is used as a sanction against permissiveness.
The more advanced and serious symptoms are emphasised
whilst the early symptoms are ignored or played down.
Precise information which is necessary for young people
to recognise the early stages of sexually transmitted

diseases if they have them, does not seem to be given.
Some of these answers to the question 'What are the
symptoms which might make you think you had VD?'
illustrate this:
  'Sores, rashes, losing your hair, leading to heart
  failure, going blind. General weakening of the body
  structure.'
The 'right' answers get confused and dramatised mainly
because the whole subject is surrounded with mystery and
horror:
  'Pains in the balls. Difficulty in urinating.
  Discharges of sperm from the penis.'
  'They show more in a man than a woman. A man - rash,
  slight greenish tinge. On a woman, violent itching,
  slight discharge.'
The way this happens would seem to be partially accounted
for by parents' attitudes to VD (see Chapter 8).
  Table 18 shows the kinds of symptoms described by boys
and girls - one in four (27%) did not know what the
symptoms were, and only 2% made reference to the difference
between male and female symptoms. A little less 'scare'
and more information might be a relevant recommendation
here.

TABLE 18   Description of venereal disease symptoms by sex

	Boys	Girls	All
	%	%	%
Discharge/pain in genital area	17	27	22
Sores, rashes, spots in genital area	24	10	17
Sores, pains, area unspecified	44	44	44
Urine problems: burning, discoloured	30	12	21
Don't know/can't say	22	32	27
Vomiting, loss of hair, heart failure, general collapse or similar extreme symptom	3	2	3
Some reference to male/female difference in symptoms	-	4	2
Never heard of VD	1	2	2
Number asked = 100%*	782	774	1,556

*   Percentages add to more than 100% because some described
    several symptoms.

YOUNG PEOPLE WHO THOUGHT THEY HAD VENEREAL DISEASE

In 1964 in Schofield's study, ten boys and five girls
were prepared to say they thought they might have had VD.
Ten years later in our study, 66 boys and 29 girls said
they thought they might have had VD at some point, that
is, 8% of the boys in the sample and 4% of the girls.
Of these young people, only 8 (3 boys and 5 girls) said
that VD had actually been diagnosed. In 1974, the
reported number of cases of gonorrhoea from 16-19-year-
olds was 11,525, that is, O.43% of the age group. If the
cases of syphilis are included, the figure rises to
O.44%. The eight reported cases of VD in our study
represent O.51% of the sample. The comparison is not
direct for three reasons: the official figures are of
cases, not individuals; any individual reporting for
treatment two or three times in one year will be counted
however many times the person is treated. Secondly, the
young people in our study who said they had had VD may
not have been treated in 1974 and thirdly, the national
rates represent cases treated in one year whereas our
figures may cover several years. Nationally, fewer boys
in the age group are treated for gonorrhoea than girls.
This is reflected in the study since more girls than boys
said they had had VD diagnosed.

Half of the boys (52%) and nearly a quarter of the
girls (24%) who thought they might have had VD did nothing
about it and reported that their symptoms disappeared.
Another 16% went to a clinic and 29% went to their general
practitioner. Twelve per cent took other courses of
action. These figures on action taken contrast with what
all the young people in the sample said they would do if
they thought they had VD. In answer to that question,
53% said they would go to their own doctor, 44% said they
would go to a VD clinic, and 1% would have asked advice
from a friend or panicked. Nobody said they would 'do
nothing and wait and see if the symptoms disappeared',
which was what nearly half (43%) of those who had thought
they had VD had done. Intentions are often coloured by
what people think they should do, and are not always
translated into action.

SUMMARY

Knowledge about the advantages and disadvantages of the
three birth control methods used most frequently by young
people (i.e., the pill, the sheath and withdrawal) seems
to be accurate when they are known, but groups of between

10% and 30%, depending on the method, said that they did
not know about the relative advantages and disadvantages.

The majority of young people who had used the pill and
the sheath gave 'correct' answers to questions about use
of these methods (85%); but more than a quarter of those
who said they had used withdrawal gave wrong answers or
said they did not know. Nearly half of those who had used
the 'safe' period failed to give correct answers, but the
numbers were small. Working-class boys were less likely
to give correct answers to these questions.

Attitudes to abortion are dominated by sex and class
variables. Boys are more likely to approve and working-
class girls are more likely to disapprove. The limited
data from the girls who had had abortions indicate that
they do use contraception, but tend to use the less
reliable methods.

Knowledge of VD is widespread but generalised. Less
than half of the young people were able to name the
symptoms. Sex education from parents and schools should
concentrate on giving detailed information, not unspeci-
fied and dramatic warnings.

4

SOURCES OF INFORMATION ABOUT
SEX AND BIRTH CONTROL

FIRST RECOLLECTIONS OF 'LEARNING' ABOUT REPRODUCTION

Learning about sex is not something which happens on one
memorable occasion. Asking these young people to describe
the way in which they first learned where babies come
from, and the age at which this happened, was, to a certain
extent, encouraging them to recall dramatic and possibly
untypical events rather than a process, which it surely
is. This seemed justifiable because the aim was to
examine sources in an attempt to illuminate the process
rather than describe the process itself. As Gagnon and
Simon point out:

> It is important to note here the extraordinary diffi-
> culties of all developmental research in getting
> accurate data and also that research on infancy and
> childhood through adulthood faces a problem which most
> of the psychoanalytic literature obscures. Part of
> the problem is faulty recall, some of which is locatable
> in the problem of inaccurate memories, but another
> source of error is located in the existentialist insight
> that instead of the past determining the character of
> the present, the present significantly reshapes the
> past as we reconstruct our biographies in an effort to
> bring them into greater congruence with our current
> identities, roles, situations and available vocabu-
> laries. (1973, p.13)

There is no way to resolve these kinds of empirical
problems satisfactorily. We would not claim, therefore,
that our findings on the way young people learned about
sex and birth control represent what actually happened,
but only what they remembered having happened at a particular stage of their development (that is, between the
age of 16 and 19). The fact that a structured questionnaire was used and the young people were interviewed for

a relatively short period means that we do not have a
considered or as full a picture as it might have been
possible to get using a different method of data collection.
In addition, the young people may have been encouraged to
remember particular events in a particular order. At the
pre-pilot and pilot stages of the research it emerged that
many young people did not remember learning or being told
about sexual intercourse at the same time as they learned
about the reproductive system. The final questionnaire
was constructed to take account of this. Care was taken,
however, not to discourage them from saying that they had
learned about reproduction and sexual intercourse at the
same time, or as a process rather than two separate events.
They were asked, 'Could you tell me how you first learned
where babies come from?', 'Could you tell me how you first
learned about sexual intercourse?', and then, 'Did you
learn about sexual intercourse at the same time as you
learned where babies come from, or did you learn about it
before or afterwards?'
    Understandably, the young people sometimes found it
difficult to remember exactly how they first learned where
babies come from:
    'I don't know. It must have been from my father,
    because I went to a convent and they were all nuns so
    they certainly didn't tell me. I suppose I just knew.
    My younger brother was born when I was about 3½ years
    old and I suppose I just started to know things from
    then on. Where the baby comes from inside the mother
    instead of from under a gooseberry bush. And I
    realised that the father had something to do with it.'
If they did have a clear picture it was sometimes obvious
that the story had been told as a family anecdote:
    'The next door neighbour was having a baby. I was four
    years old and my brother who was nine told me basic
    facts of life which I promptly forgot - so I'm told.
    I don't remember anything about it at all. The next
    door neighbour said the baby was in her stomach and I
    didn't believe her because she was always teasing me.
    I told my mother and said it couldn't be because it
    would get all mixed up with food. (WAS THIS ALL THE
    SAME DAY?) Yes. I never remembered it and when I was
    told again I didn't remember.'
However, as far as they were able to pinpoint the
occasion, two-fifths (39%) of the young people remembered
their friends as their first source of information about
reproduction (in this section reproduction is used to refer
to where babies come from) and one in four (25%) said that
one or both of their parents had been involved in that
first memory. Another 24% recalled first learning at

school from teachers. These figures show that the majority
of the young people first heard about reproduction from
their friends, their parents, or through lessons at school.
This is not a startling or unexpected finding. Most
other studies in this field have shown a similar pattern,
with friends as the most frequently mentioned source of
information (see Schofield, 1965; Gagnon and Simon, 1973).
But if comparisons are made with an earlier English study,
it seems possible that the situation is changing. Table
19 shows that compared to Schofield's findings of ten years
ago, young people are now more likely to first learn about
reproduction from their parents or from school, and less
likely to hear about it from their friends.

TABLE 19   First sources of information about reproduction
in 1964 and 1974, by sex

Source	Males		Females	
	1964	1974	1964	1974
	%	%	%	%
Friends	62	45	44	33
Parents	11	17	28	32
Teacher	12	25	18	24
Siblings	1	4	2	5
Books and media	7	12	3	13
Other sources	8	7	4	3
Don't know/can't remember	-	5	-	7
Number = 100%	934	782*	939	774*

* Percentages add to more than 100% because some young
  people mentioned more than one category as their first
  source.

This difference may be partly due to the different
questions asked in the two studies (Schofield asked, 'Who
told you about the facts of life?'), but the change could
also be said to reflect a developing awareness and
preparedness on the part of parents and teachers to tell
young people about the process of reproduction.
As the preceding table shows, there are differences in
the first sources of learning experienced by boys and
girls. Boys were more likely to hear about babies from
friends and less likely to hear from their parents than
girls. This difference is linked also to the ages at
which girls and boys first learned about reproduction, and
probably has a similar explanation.

AGE OF FIRST LEARNING ABOUT REPRODUCTION

The mean age for boys learning about reproduction was
10.3 years, and for girls, 10.0 years. The ages mentioned
ranged from five to fifteen, with a peak at eleven. One
possible explanation for girls learning about reproduction
at an earlier age than boys is that information provision
is linked to the anticipated onset of menstruation. For
boys there is no similar physical event for which they
obviously need to be prepared, and parents and teachers
may feel that it is not so necessary to tell them about
reproduction at an early age. The mean age at which both
boys and girls said they first learned about reproduction
was two years earlier than the boys and girls in Schofield's
study said they had found out about the 'facts of life'
(12.5 years for boys and 12.2 years for girls). Although
this is not a direct comparison (because of the different
questions asked), it does seem probable that children are
given, or ask for, information at an earlier age now than
ten years ago.

    This trend is backed up within our own sample with
differences between the mean age at which the younger and
older age groups said they had first learned about reproduction (9.9 years for the 16-year-olds and 10.3 years
for the 17, 18 and 19-year-olds). In spite of this
apparent trend to learning at an earlier age, over a
quarter (28%) of these 16 to 19-year-old boys and girls
did not learn about reproduction until they were 12 or
older.

    Traditionally there have been class differences in the
ways and frequency with which parents discuss sex with
their children. As Hoggart points out in his study of
the working class (1957):

    Even today few working-class parents seem to tell their
    children anything about sex.... They leave it, I think,
    partly because they are not good teachers, are neither
    competent in nor fond of exposition, prefer knowledge
    to come incidentally, by means of apophthegm and
    proverb; and partly because of this shyness about
    bringing sex to the conscious and 'sensible' level.
Although this was written twenty years ago, it seems from
our findings that it is still true. Working-class parents
are less likely to be the first remembered source of
information about babies than middle-class parents. In
this study 31% of the young people from middle-class homes
remembered their parents telling them first where babies
came from, compared with 20% of those from working-class
homes. Table 20 shows that this difference was true for
both boys and girls.

TABLE 20 First source of information on reproduction by sex and social class

Source of information	Male		Female		All
	Middle class	Working class	Middle class	Working class	
	%	%	%	%	%
Friends	38	49	31	35	39
Teachers	24	26	17	29	24
Parents	23	13	39	27	25
Books and media	13	12	11	14	13
Siblings	2	5	5	4	4
Other sources	10	5	2	4	5
Don't know/can't remember	5	4	7	6	5
Number(= 100%)*	310	431	289	427	1,556**

* Percentages add to more than 100% because some young people names more than one source.
** 41 girls and 58 boys included whose fathers' occupations were unclassified or armed forces.

The Newsons also felt that their research into child-rearing practices in Nottingham demonstrated significant differences between working-class and middle-class attitudes on 'every issue of physical or sexual modesty'. They describe two distinct 'philosophies of behaviour' in this area, attributable to the extreme ends of the social class scale. The attitude at the upper end of the scale is seen as one which engenders 'natural', 'healthy' attitudes to sex in adult life and a belief 'that a child's curiosity should be satisfied frankly and openly, and as early as his own questioning dictates'. At the other end of the scale, 'the contrasting philosophy is that sexual curiosity is suspect, sexual information dangerous and perhaps frightening for the young child, and both must be controlled by being suppressed' (1968, pp.384-6). These two philosophies, with their intervening shades, are given some substance by our findings. Table 20 shows that working-class children were less likely to say they had first been told about reproduction by their parents, and Table 21 shows that middle-class children were more likely to learn about it at an earlier age. In the sample as a whole, just over a third said they had learned first about babies before they were 10, a similar proportion had learned at the ages of 10 or 11, and just over a quarter first learned where babies come from when they were 12 or over.

TABLE 21 Age at which young people said they first learned where babies come from, by social class group

Age first learned about babies	Social Class								
	I	II	IIIn.m	IIIm.	IV	V	Armed Forces	Unclassi-fiable	All
	%	%	%	%	%	%	%	%	%
8 and under	35	29	22	18	21	21	22	18	23
9	16	15	10	10	11	8	19	22	12
10	24	17	16	21	16	15	15	8	18
11	9	20	26	19	19	17	33	13	19
12	9	11	10	13	15	21	-	21	13
13 and over	7	8	16	19	18	18	11	18	15
Mean age in years	9.4	9.6	10.2	10.5	10.4	10.5	9.8	10.3	10.2
Number (= 100%)	57	385	134	564	211	48	27	67	1,493*

* Total excludes 63 (or 4%) of the sample who could not remember when they first heard where babies come from.

LEARNING ABOUT SEXUAL INTERCOURSE

This pattern persists in the analysis of learning about
sexual intercourse. Over half (52%) of the young people
said they did not learn (or could not remember learning)
about sexual intercourse at the same time as they had
learned where babies come from.
   'I knew what it was properly when I was in about the
   2nd year of the seniors. But I didn't know properly
   and all the words and that. I sort of patched everything together, everything I knew, and I used my own
   discretion for the rest, which happened to be right
   like. I sort of matched all the pieces together.
   From talking in school like, with the older girls in
   4th year juniors. It started off with a girl talking
   about periods and then you knew babies didn't come
   from gooseberry bushes they come from your parents.
   Really and truly my friend who told me started me
   thinking, and from the end of the 4th year I'd read
   books - picked up my mother's magazines and it all
   went on from there, I pieced it all together sort of
   thing. I look at my little sister, she's 11, and she
   looks so young, and I think "Was I that young?" She
   looks too young to know anything.'
This quotation demonstrates how difficult it is to give
a definite age to the point in time when knowledge about
sexual intercourse was acquired. This and the next one
demonstrate that where babies come from was something
which had been learned separately and previously:
   'My mum told me. She was having a baby and she just
   said, "there's a baby in my stomach", sort of thing.
   She told me where babies come from, but not sort of
   how they get there, you know....'
If precise ages could not be given for the time they
learned about sexual intercourse, the lowest year age
they gave was used to calculate the mean age. Calculated
in this way, the mean age for learning about sexual intercourse was 11.6 years - over a year later than the mean
age calculated (on the same basis) for learning where
babies come from.
   One explanation for this could be that young people
are told at the same time, but the significance does not
strike them until much later, when they are told (or ask)
about sexual intercourse. On the other hand, it seems to
be common for parents and teachers to talk about reproduction without mentioning the act of intercourse.
   Amongst the group of parents interviewed in this study,
48% said they had talked to their own child about where
babies come from, but only 29% had ever talked about

sexual intercourse. Table 22 shows that fewer young people
remembered their parents as their first source of information on sexual intercourse than did for first learning
where babies come from.

TABLE 22 Proportion of boys and girls who said their
parents were their first source of information on reproduction and sexual intercourse

	Male	Female	Male and female
First learned where babies come from from parents	17%	32%	25%
First learned about sexual intercourse from parents	7%	17%	12%
Did not learn first about either from parents	83%	68%	75%
Number in sample (= 100%)	782	774	1,556

The table also shows that for both topics girls were
more likely to hear about the subject from their parents
than boys were. But only a small proportion of either
boys or girls had first learned about reproduction or
sexual intercourse from their parents.

The evidence suggests that the peer group is still the
most frequent first source of information, particularly
for boys. In a sense, it is this finding which is
probably responsible for the increase in formal sex education at school. Many adults and educators feel that it is
inappropriate for information to be given by friends, and
there is evidence too that the young people themselves
worry about it. They feel that they cannot trust the
information which comes to them from friends:

'I would have liked to learn it off my mother before
I learned off my friends because I didn't believe my
friends at first. I think when I first learned from
my friends I was under the impression that sex was
dirty and I remember hoping I wasn't born in that way
(that is, that my parents wouldn't do such a disgusting
filthy thing).'

Whilst it is true that information passed on by friends
can be disturbing and unreliable, it is also true that
they are often the only source of 'uninhibited' exchange
of sexual information and experiences. Even if all the
necessary information has been passed on by parents at an
early age, most young people will still need to discuss

this information and their own experiences with friends
in order to explore their own attitudes and feelings.

Adolescents not only have a need to know the facts
about their own bodies, its reproductive function and its
capacity for pleasure, they also need to discuss the
values and attitudes which are implicit (and often not
openly stated by parents or teachers) in the presentation
of 'facts'. The peer group allows them to do this.

Since we already know that some young people learn at
an earlier age from their parents, it is clear that not
all young people will use the peer group in the same way.
Table 23 shows that the sex and class differences shown
to exist in relation to first learning about reproduction
are maintained in relation to first learning about sexual
intercourse.

TABLE 23   First source of information on sexual intercourse
by sex and social class

Source	Male		Female		All
	Middle class	Working class	Middle class	Working class	
	%	%	%	%	%
Friends	48	51	37	34	43
Teachers	27	26	28	41	31
Parents	12	4	25	11	12
Books and media	16	14	19	18	17
Siblings	2	3	4	4	3
Other sources	9	12	5	6	7
Don't know/ can't remember	6	6	6	6	6
Number (= 100%)*	310	431	289	427	1,556**

 * Percentages add to more than 100% because some young
   people named more than one source.
** 41 boys and 58 girls included whose fathers' occupations were unclassified or armed forces.

Whilst these differences are maintained, Table 24 shows
that there is a shift in the type of first source mentioned
by all groups when the topic referred to is sexual intercourse. Both boys and girls are less likely to hear first
from their parents about sexual intercourse than they are
about reproduction, but the alternative source (on sexual
intercourse) for girls seems to be lessons at school,
whereas it is friends for boys. For both sexes there is

a small increase in the proportions first learning about
sexual intercourse from books and films. The proportion
of boys first learning about both topics at school stays
the same. Explanations for these shifts and differences
are considered in subsequent chapters.

TABLE 24   First source of information, for reproduction
and sexual intercourse, by sex

	Male		Female	
	1st source for reproduction	1st source for sexual intercourse	1st source for reproduction	1st source for sexual intercourse
	%	%	%	%
Friends	45	51	33	34
Teachers	25	26	24	37
Parents	17	7	32	17
Books and media	12	15	13	18
Siblings	4	2	5	4
Other sources	7	11	3	4
Don't know/ can't remember	5	6	7	6
Number (= 100%)*	782		774	

* Percentages add up to more than 100% because some young
  people named more than one source.

The way in which children first hear about reproduction
needs to be set in context of their previous and subsequent
experience. They do not suddenly hear the 'facts' about
reproduction at the age of 7, 10 or 12 in a vacuum. The
actual details of fertilisation and intercourse may not be
known and may come as a surprise to some, but all children
are aware of their genitalia and the differences in appear-
ances of boys and girls. This physiological knowledge is
not, in the early stages, equated with sexual knowledge.
As Plummer points out in his book 'Sexual Stigma' (1975,
p.30), 'Nothing is sexual but naming makes it so.... This
is not, of course, to deny the existence of genitals,

TABLE 25   People with whom teenagers had discussed specific topics

Topic	Mother %	Father %	Male friend %	Female friend %	Male teacher %	Female teacher %	Elder sister %	Elder brother %	Spouse %	Fiancé (e) %	Doctor %	Other person %
Animal reproduction	10	7	20	19	15	16	5	4	2	2	1	8
Human reproduction	35	16	43	43	17	20	12	8	4	5	3	18
Sexual intercourse	34	16	66	63	17	18	14	11	5	6	9	22
Female puberty	37	10	37	43	14	17	12	6	3	3	7	17
Male puberty	18	11	32	31	13	14	7	6	3	3	2	11
Family and parenthood	35	20	31	39	13	14	12	7	4	5	4	15
Personal relationships	33	17	50	54	14	14	13	8	4	5	4	19

TABLE 25   Continued

Topic	Mother %	Father %	Male friend %	Female friend %	Male teacher %	Female teacher %	Elder sister %	Elder brother %	Spouse %	Fiancé (e) %	Doctor %	Other person %
Mastur-bation	7	4	37	27	7	6	5	5	3	3	1	8
Abortion	34	13	44	53	12	14	13	7	4	5	3	16
Homo-sexuality	15	8	43	36	9	8	8	7	3	3	1	11
Lesbianism	14	6	38	36	8	7	7	6	3	3	1	10
Venereal Disease	23	10	48	43	14	15	9	8	3	4	4	13

Number (= 100%)*   1,556

* Percentages add to more than 100% because many young people named more than one subject.

copulation or orgasms as biological and universal "facts",
it is simply to assert the sociological commonplace that
these things do not have "sexual meanings" in their own
right.' We did not explore levels of sexual awareness or
knowledge before the point at which the young people
recalled first learning about reproduction, and are unable
therefore to discuss the context in which the young people
first heard about reproduction. But it was possible to
look at the sources of information about sex which
followed the initial source. This means that the subsequent pattern of exposure to information can be examined.
It does not mean that statements can be made about
sexuality or about sexual knowledge received and retained.
To some extent, what the individual defines as sexual
knowledge is acquired, not only through information
received, but also through personal experiences and
observations of other people's behaviour. In this sense,
the study has important gaps. But since information is an
integral part of learning and acquired knowledge it would
seem to be important to know how that knowledge is
acquired. As Plummer points out (1975, p.58):

> For many groups, the most important stage of building
> up sexual meanings will be that of adolescence - a
> time when past unnamed 'sexual' encounters may be
> retrospectively interpreted, and a stable sexual world
> view allowed to emerge. A number of significant others
> will influence what takes place at this stage - isolated
> self-interaction, concrete peer interaction and
> generalised media interaction are three crucially
> important ones.

Although the first of these situations was not fully
explored in this study (Plummer is referring mainly to
masturbation) because of the practical difficulties
involved, masturbation was found to be one of the topics
least frequently discussed with all informants, including
friends. Table 25 shows which topics had been discussed
with particular people.

Friends emerge here quite clearly as the people all
topics had been discussed with most frequently. Female
puberty and family and parenthood were the two topics
discussed as frequently with mothers as with friends.
Whilst it is obvious that many young people had discussed
a range of sex-related topics with a number of people, a
few (1%) said that they had not talked about any of the
topics mentioned with anyone.

This emphasis on friends continues when the most
frequent source of discussion and the people found to be
most helpful for learning about sex are explored. Over
half the boys (59%) gave male friends as the person they

had talked to most often about sex, and one in three girls
(31%) mentioned a group of other girlfriends. Mothers
were the next most frequently mentioned person for girls
(28%) but were followed by one girlfriend, who was
mentioned as the person 25% of the girls had talked to
most often about sex. Most discussions about sex apparently take place between members of the same sex when the
people talking are girls, but boys mentioned girlfriends
as the people they talked to most often after a group of
male friends (19% said this) and one male friend was the
most common confidant for 15% of the boys. Boys maintained their dependence on other male friends when they
were asked who they felt had been the most helpful person
when it came to learning about sex, but mothers moved to
the top of the list for girls. Table 26 shows this, and
the fact that middle-class boys were more likely to say
that no one person had been more helpful than another,
than working-class boys were. Middle-class girls were
also more likely than working-class girls to say that
female friends and one male friend had been the most
helpful person they had talked to.

TABLE 26 Who was most helpful in learning about sex by
sex and social class

	MALES		FEMALES		
	Middle class	Working class	Middle class	Working class	All
	%	%	%	%	%
Mother	9	6	19	22	14
Father	5	3	2	1	3
Male friend	7	10	13	7	9
Female friend	8	8	11	12	9
Male friends	20	22	1	1	11
Female friends	3	4	13	7	7
Male teacher	8	9	2	2	5
Female teacher	2	3	5	9	5
Older sister	1	1	6	8	4
Older brother	3	4	–	–	2
Spouse or fiancé(e)	2	2	6	9	5
Other	4	4	5	8	5
No one person more helpful	20	14	15	10	14
No-one helpful	5	7	1	3	5
Not talked	3	3	1	1	2
Number of young people (=100%)	310	431	289	427	1,556*

* 99 included whose fathers' occupations were unclassified
  or armed forces.

It is clear from these findings that friends represent the most frequent source of information and verbal contact about sex for young people, particularly for boys. Later chapters show that this is not always regarded as a satis- factory state of affairs. The sex differences in initial and subsequent sources override class differences, which do exist in the earlier stages of learning but tend to disappear later on.

BOOKS AND MEDIA

As shown earlier (in Tables 20 and 23) books and films about reproduction and sexual intercourse were said to be the first source of information for 13% and 17% of the young people. It was relatively unusual, however, for books or films to be the first single source of informa- tion. For this reason, and because this source does not have a chapter devoted to it, as do parents, friends and schools, the discussion which follows is in greater detail.

Of those who mentioned them as a first source for learning where babies come from, 43% had used books or seen films as part of sex education lessons at school, and the same was true for 35% of those who said that they were one of their first sources of information on sexual intercourse. In some cases, films seem to have represen- ted the sum total of a sex education lesson, but because films were seen or books read in a lesson context, they cannot be viewed in the same way as those who simply took books from a library or read them at home alone. Only 3% of the teenagers named books as their only source of information when they first learned about reproduction, but 6% said this was the way they first learned about sexual intercourse.

Books were a much more frequent source of information after the initial learning stage, and nearly two-thirds (62%) of the young people said that they had read books or articles about sexual matters at some stage. The most frequently mentioned sources were women's magazines (15%) and sex magazines like Forum, Penthouse and Mayfair (15%). Other written sources mentioned included biology books (8%) and psychology books (9%), novels and other magazines (10%), and pamphlets about specific topics like VD and abortion and birth control (4%). Because of the diffi- culties of remembering and defining literature with a sex information content, these figures probably under-represent the amount of information young people do come across in written sources. But for those who could remember reading

such material, friends again played an important part in
its provision. A third of the young people (39%) said
that what they had read had been given to them by friends,
a third (31%) said that they had bought the books for
themselves, or in the case of pamphlets had written away
for them. Other sources included parents or finding
books at home (21%) and libraries (13%).

Reactions to these written sources of information on
reproduction and sex were not over-enthusiastic. Only
one in four of those who had remembered reading something
said that it had been very helpful (21%). The rest said
that it had been fairly helpful or not very helpful at
all. Working-class boys were more likely than any others
to say that the literature they had seen had not been
very helpful (36% compared with 32% of middle-class boys,
28% of middle-class girls, and 18% of working-class girls).

Television is a potentially influential source of
information for young people, and it is perhaps surprising
that so few of them mentioned it as a first source. On
the other hand, so much of television could be classified
as 'sexual information' that it is not unlikely that the
teenagers could simply not recall specific information
which they had gathered from this source in their early
years. In the later stages, however, television became
a more frequently mentioned source. A third of the young
people (35%) said they had seen at least one programme on
television about sex or related topics (22% of them
mentioned a documentary programme which they had
remembered seeing and 13% just remembered unspecific
programmes). Again, their reactions to these films were
unenthusiastic, with the majority (77%) of those who had
seen them saying that they had found them fairly useful
or not very useful as a source of information.

Although in themselves books and films are not
apparently a primary (or preferred) source of information
for young people, they should not be seen as irrelevant
to the learning process but rather as an aid to be used
in conjunction with other more personal sources. This is
particularly true for learning about birth control.

LEARNING ABOUT BIRTH CONTROL

Opinions vary about the relevant stage at which young
people should be given information about birth control.
Parents may often be torn between their desire to protect
their children's 'innocence' and the need to ensure that
they know how to protect themselves from unwanted
pregnancy if and when they become sexually active. The

Newsons (1968, pp.385-6) point out that parents of both
classes are 'agreed that the child's sexual innocence,
better termed sexual naiveté, should be preserved' and
that it is only the ways in which they choose to protect
this innocence that the classes differ. Most of the
parents interviewed in this study agreed that young people
should be told about birth control (92%) at some stage.
The ages at which they felt it appropriate for this
information to be given varied from before they were 10
to after they were 17, but the mean age they gave when
asked what age young people should learn about birth
control was 13.1 years for girls and 13.7 years for boys.
Also, half of the parents (49%) felt that young people
should be told 'everything' about birth control, including
a full description of individual methods. Ideally then,
most of the parents interviewed for this study were in
favour of detailed birth control information being given
at a reasonably early age. Whether they considered themselves to be an appropriate source of information and
whether they had told their own children is discussed in
Chapter 6.

Sources

Friends were again registered as the most common point of
reference when talking about birth control. Two out of
every three teenagers (68%) said they had talked to one
female friend about it, and 61% said they had discussed
birth control with a male friend. There are differences
within the types of peer group referred to by boys and
girls. Boys consistently named other boys throughout the
three levels of talking to, talking to most often, and
the person most helpful. Table 27 shows this, and also
the fact that for girls, mothers supported or took the
place of the peer group in the 'talked to most often'
and 'found most helpful' categories. The only 'outsider'
(i.e. non-peer grouper) for boys is the male teacher, who
ranks third in the list of people most helpful to talk to
about birth control. This pattern follows quite closely
the one established in sources about reproduction with
the additional introduction of teachers for boys.

TABLE 27   Groups and people teenagers discussed birth
control with in order mentioned most often

	MALES	%	FEMALES	%
Talked to	Male friends	71	One female friend	80
ever about	One male friend	70	Female friends	69
birth	One female friend	56	Mother	62
control	Female friends	41	One male friend	51
Talked to	Male friends	38	Female friends	24
most often	One female friend	14	One female friend	20
about birth	One male friend	12	Mother	17
control	Female friends	9	One male friend	16
Found most	Male friends	19	Mother	15
helpful to	Male teacher	8	Female friends	14
talk to	One female friend	8	One female friend	13
about birth	One male friend	7	Doctor	9
control				
Number				
(= 100%)		782		774

Parents

Although mothers were mentioned most frequently by girls
as the person they had found most helpful to talk to about
birth control, overall she represents the second most
frequently mentioned discussion source (after friends).
Altogether, 47% of the young people said that they had,
at some time, talked to their mothers about birth control,
with twice as many girls as boys saying this was so (62%
of the girls had talked to their mothers compared with 31%
of the boys). Father figures less prominently, with only
18% of young people saying they had ever discussed birth
control with him. The sex differences were reversed here,
as might be expected, with 24% of the boys saying they had
talked to their fathers and only 13% of the girls. Unlike
mothers, fathers did not feature at all in the list of
people the teenagers said they had found most helpful to
talk to about birth control. Only 2% named fathers as
their most useful source.

Lessons at school

Over half the teenagers in this study (58%) said they had
never been told about birth control in school. But 42% of

boys and girls said that the subject had been discussed
in lessons. In the third follow-up of the National Child
Development Study (Fogelman, 1976, p.42), 55% of 16-year-
olds attended schools which said they provided lessons on
birth control. The number of 16-year-olds in our study
who said they had had birth control lessons was 50%, which
reflects quite closely the proportion of schools saying
they provided birth control information in the National
Child Development Study. The average age at which young
people had had the lessons was 14.2 years, and the difference between the mean age for boys and girls was the
reverse of the difference between the ages they had first
learned about reproduction. There the findings suggest
that girls learn before boys; with birth control, boys
learn at an earlier age than girls, 14.0 years compared
with 14.4 years.

SUMMARY

A trend to earlier learning about reproduction is apparent
when comparisons are made with Schofield's findings of
twelve years ago. There is little doubt that friends are
the most frequently mentioned source of information on
reproduction, sexual intercourse and birth control, both
at the initial and subsequent stages of learning. They
are also named more frequently than parents or teachers
as the most helpful person in the learning process.
Comparison with an earlier study suggests that this
situation may be changing and that parents and teachers
are more often the first source of information now than
they were twelve years ago.
    Sources of information seem to change with the topic.
This may be because adults are reluctant to discuss the
more intimate subjects like intercourse and masturbation,
or because they do not realise that their children (or
pupils) are ready to learn about these things. It is
also possible that young people avoid discussions of such
topics with adults because they do not feel they are an
appropriate source. Books and films are not often
mentioned as a single first source of information, nor
are they viewed over-enthusiastically as a helpful source
of information. It seems likely that they are seen and
used as an aid to learning, rather than a primary source.

5

WHAT DID MOTHER SAY?

Little is known about the way in which parents tell their
children about sex, how much information they give them,
or at what stages in their development. The role of the
family as an agent of socialisation has been explored
by many sociologists (Parsons and Bales, 1955; Bell and
Vogel, 1961; Coser, 1974; Morgan, 1975), and it is
obvious that parental attitudes to sex and sexual matters
will be an important factor in the development of their
children's attitudes. In this chapter, the aim is simply
to describe the kinds of information the young people in
our study said they received from their mothers and
fathers, the age they were when they were given it, and
how they felt about it. The analysis and interpretation
of the relationship of parents' attitudes and information
to the sexual attitudes and behaviour of young people is
discussed in Chapter 7.

In the preceding chapter it emerged that parents were
the second most frequently mentioned source of information
on reproduction and sexual intercourse at the initial
stages. Later in the learning process their frequency as
a source of information varied with the topic. Reproduction (where babies come from) was the subject most
often discussed by parents. Whilst 24% of young people
said their mother or father had been the first person to
tell them about babies, nearly two-thirds of the group
(63%) said that they had discussed this subject with
either one or both parents at some stage. The proportions
who had ever discussed sexual intercourse with their
parents was lower at 38%, and half (50%) the teenagers had
talked about birth control to their parents.

Chapter 4 also showed that girls were more likely than
boys to learn first about reproduction and sexual intercourse from their parents. They were also more likely to
have discussed reproduction and sexual intercourse with

their parents at later stages. Nearly two-thirds of the girls (61%) had discussed where babies come from with their parents, and 43% had talked about sexual intercourse. These two subjects had been discussed with parents at some stage by 37% and 33% of the boys. This means that nearly two-thirds of the boys (60%) had never discussed either topic with their parents. One possible explanation for this different treatment of boys and girls is the difference in pubertal development. Menstruation is a positive event which needs preparation, even if it is simply in terms of the use of sanitary towels. For boys there is no similar happening, and changes in their physiology are easier to ignore, partly because they happen gradually and partly because they are not so obviously connected to the reproductive system. It seemed appropriate, therefore, to look at the relationship between the way girls learned about menstruation, reproduction and sexual intercourse.

LEARNING ABOUT PERIODS

Often one of the dramatic events in a girl's early life happens when she begins her periods. There is little available evidence to show how many mothers tell their daughters about periods or at what stage girls are prepared for it. In a study of 11 and 12-year-old girls from a Lancashire town, Leeson and Stein (1964) found that nearly a third of them had or were approaching the menarche without having been prepared for it by their mothers. The proportion is similar in our study, where 66% of the girls said that their mothers had told them about periods, but of the rest, 32% had learned from other people and 2% said no one had told them. If they had been told by their mothers they were less likely to have been told before they began their periods (66% of girls told before the event were told by mothers, compared with 86% told afterwards). In fact, the majority of girls (86%) had been told about menstruation before it happened to them, 5% were told at the same time as they began their periods, 7% were told afterwards, and 2% said they had never been told. The average age at which the girls were told about menstruation was 10.8 years.

'I didn't [learn]. I was frightened and ran to Mum and said, "Mum, I can't stop bleeding." She just told me this was what girls had to have. She told me that now I mustn't go near boys or do this or that - I was scared to even look at a boy in case I got pregnant.'

The average age at which these girls had started to menstruate was 12.5 years, almost two years after they had

been told about the event. So the group as a whole were
apparently prepared for menstruation well in advance. In
looking for an explanation why some girls were told after
their periods began, one possibility is that these were
the girls who started their periods at an earlier age,
before their mothers expected it. As Leeson and Stein
(1964) point out: 'Mothers are uncertain whether the
school will take on a responsibility which they themselves
find hard to fulfil. In the meantime, some girls begin to
menstruate before anyone has accepted the responsibility'.
Our findings suggest that this is so. The girls who were
told before they began their periods, began to menstruate
at a mean age of 12.6 years, compared with a mean age of
11.9 years for those girls who were not told until after
they began their periods.

Girls whose mothers had educational qualifications were
more likely to have learned about periods before they
began and to have learned at an earlier age (92% of girls
with 'qualified' mothers learned about periods before they
began, compared with 84% of girls with 'unqualified'
mothers; girls with 'qualified' mothers learned about
periods at a mean age of 10.4 years, compared with 10.8
years for girls with 'unqualified' mothers (t = 3.07)).
The mean age of menstruation, however, was 12.5 years for
both girls with 'qualified' mothers and girls with mothers
who had no educational qualifications. The findings on
social class differences reflect these results since,
although the girls from middle-class homes were on average
younger when they learned about periods, they did not
begin their periods at an earlier age than girls from
working-class families. This finding is consistent with
those from other post-war studies which show that although
the age of menarche is related to physical maturity, the
class differences in height and weight which existed before
the war have decreased (see Roberts and Dann, 1975;
Douglas, 1966).

If average ages of learning about reproduction, periods
and sexual intercourse reflect a general pattern, then it
seems that girls learn first about reproduction and babies,
then about menstruation usually during the early part of
their eleventh year. Between the ages of 11 and 13 they
learn about sexual intercourse and begin their periods.
It seems likely that early sex education from mothers to
daughters might sometimes be linked to the anticipated
event of the menarche. However, there is no significant
correlation between the age of menstruation and the age at
which they learn about sexual intercourse. Amongst the
mothers we interviewed, only 6 (that is, 6%) said that
they had never discussed periods with their daughters, but

a further 19 (20%) admitted that the discussion had
taken place after the event. Altogether, less than half
the mothers (43%) said that they had initiated these
discussions with their daughters, and a third (33%) said
that it had been the daughter who had raised the subject.

Other sources of information about periods

Although nearly all the girls had, at some time, talked
to their mothers about menstruation, only two-fifths of
them (41%) had first learned about this 'female fact of
life' in a talk with their mothers. What they had learned,
of course, varied from:
  'I think my mother just said if we ever had any blood
  in our knickers to tell her. We didn't really understand it.'
to:
  'I was told that along with everything else by my
  mother before I went to [secondary] school.'
Altogether then, just over half (55%) had first learned
in some way from their mothers. The remaining 45% first
learned from a variety of sources, including friends,
siblings, school teachers, and from the experience of
beginning their periods. The majority of girls who had
learned from their mothers expressed satisfaction about
the way they had learned:
  'I think I was just dying to have one because I was
  one of the last in my class. I certainly wasn't
  upset or worried about it. I remember being slightly
  bemused by it being called "the curse" for the first
  year when I had it because I was so thrilled.'
Altogether, three-fifths (60%) of the girls who first
learned from their mothers said that they were satisfied
with the way they learned, compared with a third (32%) of
those who learned from sources other than their mother,
or just picked it up:
  'I'd have liked to have been told proper, sat down
  and had a talk about it instead of finding out in bits
  and pieces. I knew you bled from somewhere but where
  I didn't know. I was shocked, I didn't know what was
  happening. It would have helped me if I'd been told.'
  'I don't think I learned the right way. I'd rather
  my Mum had told me.'
On the other hand, a small group (17%) who had been
told by their mothers had criticisms of the way they had
learned, and some of the girls who recalled other sources
(32%) expressed satisfaction with the way they had learned:
  'I'm glad I had it from my mates rather than being
  taken aside by anyone.'

But most of the girls who were satisfied with the way
they had learned, if they had not been told by their
mothers, had learned from lessons at school:
 'I was satisfied really. We had a lecture and then
 we had a booklet and it was all very clear, and I wasn't
 embarrassed or frightened about starting or anything
 like that.'
Clearly, satisfaction with the way girls had learned about
periods is linked to whether they had been told by what
they regarded as an authoritative source - mother first
and teacher second.

Boys learning about menstruation

Although it is obvious that boys do not need to be told
about periods for the same reasons as girls, they do need
to be told about their own pubertal development, and
ideally also about changes in girls' bodies, including
menstruation. Relatively few boys had ever discussed
male puberty with either their mother or father (17% and
16% respectively) so this was not a topic used to lead
into reproduction. Neither, it seems, was menstruation
widely discussed within the family. Only one in ten boys
had been told about girls having periods by their mothers,
and even fewer by their fathers (3%). The boys who had
not been told by their parents learned either at school
(33%) or from their friends (29%). One in four of the
boys said that they had never been told that girls had
periods, but had learned indirectly by hearing their
friends chat about it (12%), from books or articles (7%),
and the rest from an assortment of girlfriends, sisters,
brothers and jokes.
 Amongst the mothers and fathers interviewed in this
study, only 14% of the mothers and 18% of the fathers
said they had talked to their sons about girls having
periods, and in one in every three of these cases the
subject had been raised by the son. Five per cent of
the fathers said they had not discussed this with their
sons because it was something they left to their wives.
A third of the fathers (37%) said the matter had never
cropped up. Another group (37%) said it had not been
necessary because their sons already knew, and the rest
(21%) said they would have been embarrassed or could not
say why they had not discussed it.
 Mothers who said they had not discussed it with their
sons said it had not occurred to them to do so, or if it
had they said they would have been embarrassed:
 'I'm just hoping he knows from being taught at school.
 It's different with a boy - if he'd been a girl I'd
 have said, I think.'

Several fathers expressed the opinion that it was
wholly a female concern and therefore nothing to do with
them:
   'Having three boys in the family, monthly periods have
   never arisen - we've never even had a bitch - it's
   always been a dog. In fact, we don't know much about
   females in this family.'

TOPICS IN FOCUS

In terms of the three topics most relevant to the early
stages of learning about sex within the family, where
babies come from, sexual intercourse and menstruation,
boys are less likely to be told by their parents and less
likely ever to discuss these subjects at any stage with
them. The mother-daughter relationship is the important
factor, although mothers are more likely to discuss the
subjects with their sons than fathers are. Although it
seems likely that in some cases the subject of menstruation may prompt discussions about sexual intercourse
between mothers and daughters, the fact that girls learn
about 'babies' first, then menstruation, followed by
sexual intercourse, indicates that the 'mother' role is
the first component of sexuality to be passed on to or
learned by them, within the family. Of course, this is
not always true, since 34% of the girls remembered
learning about babies and sexual intercourse at the same
time. Those girls who had discussed both subjects with
their mothers were more likely to have learned about
reproduction and sexual intercourse at the same time.
This was also true for the few boys who had discussed
these subjects with their parents.

LEARNING ABOUT BIRTH CONTROL WITHIN THE FAMILY

Birth control was not talked about in the family as
frequently as reproduction, but had been discussed
between parents and children more frequently than sexual
intercourse. Altogether, half (50%) of the young people
said that they had talked to either one or both of their
parents about birth control, but once again the mother-
daughter discussion was more common than either the
mother-son or father-son talk. Nearly two-thirds of the
girls (62%) and a third (31%) of the boys had discussed
birth control with their mothers. Fathers were reported
to have been involved in discussions with 24% of the boys
and 13% of the girls.

Birth control is a different kind of topic from
reproduction, in that it involves the practical application of technical knowledge. Perhaps reflecting this
difference, only 18% of the young people felt that
learning from parents was the best way to learn about
birth control, whereas 37% had felt that parents were the
best source of information for learning about sex. Many
of the young people felt that if parents did tell their
children about birth control they would need some help,
either from an 'expert' or from a written source:
'I think parents should explain and get pamphlets for
us and explain them to us.'
'I think parents should tell you first and then some
special kind of person who knows more about it.'
Some definitely excluded parents from the business of
learning about birth control:
'From someone who knows about it. Your doctor or
someone like that who knows more about it than your
parents.'
More parents than young people thought that they should
be the ones to tell children about birth control: 35% of
the mothers and 29% of the fathers said that parents
telling children was the best way for young people to
learn about birth control. However, for some fathers this
would appear to be more of an ideal than a reality, since
only 15% had actually discussed birth control with their
own children. The mothers seemed to have carried out
their ideals because 37% of them had talked to their own
children about birth control, although only a third of
these had initiated the discussions.
In a way it is reassuring that the majority of young
people and parents do not see the family as the best
source of information on birth control. This is particularly so when parents' knowledge of birth control is
considered. Nearly half the parents (44%) admitted that
they had not heard of all the methods of birth control.
One mother said she had not heard of the pill. Table 28
shows which methods the mothers and fathers said they knew
nothing about or had not heard of. These findings are
similar to those in a study carried out in 1968
(Cartwright, 1970, p.28), where 10% of mothers had not
heard of the cap and the IUD was the least well known of
the three medically prescribed methods.

TABLE 28   Parents' knowledge of birth control methods

Methods of birth control parents said they had not heard of	Mothers	Fathers
	%	%
Pill	1	-
IUD	7	12
Cap	9	11
Sheath	4	2
Chemicals	42	35
Withdrawal	7	4
Safe period	8	4
Male sterilisation	4	1
Female sterilisation	3	1
Heard of all these methods	54	61
Number = 100%*	184**	160**

 * Percentages add to more than 100% because some parents
   had heard of only a few methods.
** 2 mothers and 3 fathers excluded because inadequate
   answers.

SOCIAL CLASS

Alongside the different pattern of learning about sex and
birth control for boys and girls within the family, and
the way different topics are approached by parents, there
are also social class differences. These really bear out
the findings in Chapter 4, that middle-class children
were more likely to have learned first of all from their
parents, and were also more likely to have ever discussed
all the topics with their parents. As expected, the
characteristics of those young people who had discussed
reproduction and sexual intercourse with their parents are
different from those who never had. Those who said neither
parent had ever told them about babies or sexual intercourse were more likely to be the children of manual
workers, more likely to be working and not in full-time
education, and less likely to have parents with educational qualifications. Only 26% of manual workers'
children said they had been told about both reproduction
and sexual intercourse by either parent, compared with
38% of non-manual workers' children. Of those who were
working, 73% said their parents had never told them about

babies or sexual intercourse compared with 61% of those who were still at school or college. Finally, 27% of those whose parents did not have educational qualifications had been told compared with 43% of those young people whose parents did have educational qualifications.

The pattern is repeated where birth control discussions within the family are concerned when 50% of middle-class teenagers had discussed birth control with their mothers compared with 44% of working-class teenagers, and 25% of middle-class teenagers with their fathers compared with 14% of those whose fathers had manual occupations.

In spite of the feeling constantly being expressed that parents are the 'best' people to teach their children about sex, this chapter throws some doubt on whether this is necessarily and always the case. Not enough thought has been given to the problems faced by both parents and children in this area. Gagnon and Simon point to one of the greatest difficulties involved when they say:

For parents to take on the serious responsibility for the sex education of their children...would immediately involve having to present a sense of their own sexuality to their children and, at the same time, admit to themselves the sexual nature of their children. For the majority of adults it is difficult to conceive of a way in which this can be done without provoking the most profound ambivalences on the part of the child, and equally profound anxieties on the part of the parent. (1973, p.117)

The next chapter illustrates this parental ambivalence amongst the mothers and fathers interviewed in this study.

6

PARENTS' BELIEFS AND ACTIONS

This chapter looks at the popular assumption that parents are the right people to tell children about reproduction and sex. It also shows the extent to which some parents carry out their beliefs, and looks at the obstacles and difficulties they encountered.

Although there are no directly comparable English studies, there is some evidence which suggests that parents feel they should tell their children about reproduction (Gill, Reid and Smith, 1974), but that some experience difficulty in doing so. The Newsons (1968, pp.346-88) explain parental reluctance to discuss sex with their offspring in terms of embarrassment and difficulty in communicating their feelings:

> The practical outcome in terms of the training process is that parents expect children to obey the principles of modesty while at the same time they object to making those principles explicit. Over and above this, for large numbers of parents in our culture, failure to communicate goes much deeper, in that they feel a positive embarrassment about discussing with their children *any* aspect of sex.

This 'embarrassment' is explained slightly differently by Gagnon and Simon (1973) when they point to the difficulties parents experience in talking to their children about sex because it involves presenting 'a sense of their own sexuality'. Freudian psychologists and the structural functionalist sociologists (see Parsons and Bales, 1955, pp.98-104) consider that some of the difficulties are related to the incest taboo: 'The incest taboo then means, not only that erotic attachment within the nuclear family is repressed, but its revival is permitted *only* outside the nuclear family.'

This chapter illustrates that to a large extent the parents we talked to did see themselves as sex educators

but, for a variety of reasons, had often failed to carry
out the task.

PARENTS' VIEWS OF WHO SHOULD TELL BOYS AND GIRLS ABOUT
REPRODUCTION AND SEXUAL INTERCOURSE

Nearly all the parents felt, in principle, that either
they or their spouses should be the first people to tell
their children about reproduction (the parents were asked:
'Do you think boys/girls should first be told where babies
come from by their: mother, father, teacher, friends,
someone else, or no-one?'). Immediately it is clear that
mothers take, and are expected by fathers to take, a more
active role in preparing young people for this aspect of
adulthood. The data show that twice as many mothers felt
that they should do the telling and twice as many fathers
said that mothers should be the first person to tell the
child than felt they should be involved. The majority of
those parents who did not nominate either one or both
parents said that they thought teachers should be the
first to do the telling (28%), and a few (3%) said that
no-one should actually tell children about babies.

TABLE 29   Who should first tell about babies

Who should first tell boys/girls where babies come from	Mothers	Fathers	All
	%	%	%
Mother	61	67	64
Father	30	30	30
Other person	36	31	34
Should not be told	3	3	3
Number = 100%*	186	163	349

* Percentages add to more than 100% because some parents
  mentioned more than one source.

   Fewer parents felt that they should be the first
people to tell about sexual intercourse (they were asked:
'Do you think that boys/girls should first be told about
sexual intercourse by their: mother, father, teacher,
friends, someone else or no-one?'), and more of them
mentioned teachers for this topic than had for where
babies come from. It is clear from the data that fewer
mothers felt that they were the most appropriate source
for this topic, and fewer fathers named mothers as the

person who should tell about sexual intercourse. A few
more fathers nominated themselves for the task than had
done for telling about babies, but in the main, those who
felt that sexual intercourse was not an appropriate topic
for parents to discuss named teachers as the people to
give information. The reasons given by the parents who
felt no one should tell children about sexual intercourse
were a mixture of apprehension:
>'Most kids don't ask. The idea of sitting them down
>and telling them is a load of rubbish...if you know
>theory then you're going to practise.'

and the feeling that it was something which they would
become aware of:
>'Too much is made of it - it needn't be put formally
>to them.'

TABLE 30   Who should first tell children about sexual
intercourse

Who should first tell boys/girls about sexual intercourse	Mothers	Fathers	All
	%	%	%
Mother	48	55	51
Father	32	35	33
Other person	41	36	39
Should not be told	6	4	5
Number = 100%*	186	163	349

* Percentages add to more than 100% because some mentioned
more than one source.

Mothers and fathers, sons and daughters

Earlier chapters suggested that mothers were reported as
having been involved in telling about sex and as having
been most helpful more frequently than fathers. This
section looks at the parents' own feelings about their own
and their spouses' roles. When the findings are analysed
into groups: mothers and sons, mothers and daughter,
fathers and sons, and fathers and daughters; the numbers
are small, and the sample is biased in certain ways (see
Appendix III). We cannot claim therefore that these
views are necessarily representative of all parents.
However, the findings do suggest that mothers and fathers
see their own and each other's roles differently and that
this perception varies with the sex of the child.

TABLE 31 Who should first tell about reproduction and sexual intercourse by sex of 'key' child and sex of parent

Who should first tell	First telling about babies				First telling about sexual intercourse			
	Mothers asked about daughters	Fathers asked about daughters	Mothers asked about sons	Fathers asked about sons	Mothers asked about daughters	Fathers asked about daughters	Mothers asked about sons	Fathers asked about sons
	%	%	%	%	%	%	%	%
Mother alone	60	60	18	24	52	53	5	11
Both parents	12	16	21	30	12	12	10	27
Father alone	-	-	15	6	-	1	29	18
Parents with others	7	4	9	5	10	6	14	7
Teachers alone	18	12	25	30	16	18	29	25
Others alone	-	5	10	2	3	7	9	7
No-one should tell	3	3	2	3	7	3	4	5
Number = 100%	95	74	91	89	94*	74	91	88*

* 2 answers to this question were inadequate.

Table 31 shows that a sex-related parent-child pattern
of beliefs emerges for telling about reproduction. (The
mothers and fathers were asked all these questions in
relation to either boys or girls. The decision as to
which sex child they were asked about was made by the
interviewer on the basis of the principles described in
Appendix III.) More mothers expected and were expected
by fathers to be involved in first telling girls where
babies come from and about sexual intercourse. Neither
mothers nor fathers thought that fathers should give the
information alone to girls. Their expectations are less
straightforward where boys are concerned. Fewer mothers
than fathers felt that mothers alone should be involved
in the first telling (although the difference was not
significant), and relatively small numbers of fathers
wanted to carry out the task alone. Both mothers and
fathers seemed to move towards shared telling for boys on
the subject of reproduction, but more mothers expected
the responsibility for telling boys about sexual intercourse to be taken by fathers on their own (although
again the difference was not significant). This is a
possible explanation for why fewer boys are told about
sex by their parents, because parents do not agree about
their respective roles. Their disagreement possibly
resolves itself in this context by the shelving of
discussions or by the shifting of responsibility to
teachers. Larger proportions of both mothers and fathers
said that teachers alone should be the first person to
tell boys about reproduction and sexual intercourse.

Social class

Differences in the way middle-class and working-class
parents believe young people should be told about reproduction emerged in line with the differences reported by
the young people. Other studies which have looked at
this subject (Newsons, 1968; Douglas, 1964; Gill, Reid
and Smith, 1974) suggest that middle-class parents are
more likely to think that they should talk to their
children and answer their questions than working-class
parents. This was true in our study, but only for first
telling about babies. For sexual intercourse, similar
proportions believed that parents should tell first,
although the working-class preference for teachers
remained.
Table 32 shows the proportions of parents in each
social class who thought particular people should be
involved in first telling children about reproduction.

Almost the same proportions of working-class parents thought they should be involved in telling children about both topics, but middle-class parents apparently felt more reluctant or felt it less appropriate that they should be the first ones to tell children about sexual intercourse. Of those middle-class parents who thought parents should tell children about 'babies' but not about sexual inter-course (9%), the majority thought teachers should be the ones to tell about sexual intercourse, and a few (1%) thought that no one should tell them. It might have been expected, given the work on joint conjugal roles (Bott, 1957; and Rainwater, 1965), that middle-class parents would be more likely to believe that this was a task they should do together. But these kinds of class differences do not seem to exist in relation to talking to their children about sex.

TABLE 32 Parents' beliefs about who should tell children about reproduction and sexual intercourse, by social class

Who should tell first	Where babies come from		Sexual intercourse	
	Middle class	Working class	Middle class	Working class
	%	%	%	%
Mother alone	45	35	34	28
Both parents	20	20	19	11
Father alone	6	5	7	16
Others and parents	2	1	2	1
Teacher and parents	6	4	9	8
Teacher alone	13	29	19	26
Others alone	7	3	8	3
No-one should tell	1	3	2	7
Number = 100%	142	184	140*	183*

* 2 middle-class parents and 1 working-class parent gave
  inadequate answers to this question.

   Class differences also emerged in respect of the stage at which young people should be told about sex. The timing at which information is given can often determine its usefulness to young people. Since many young people seemed to expect their parents to tell them about these things, and since the range of potential sources of information increases as adolescence approaches, parents'

views on the appropriate age for telling about reproduction
and sexual intercourse are important. Parents and teachers
may feel that they should be careful not to 'spoil' childhood by giving explicit information about sexuality before
it is necessary. Uncertainty or unawareness of development may mean that they leave it 'too late' in the sense
that misleading or confusing information has already been
passed on from friends. One mother said, reflecting the
feeling that 11 was too early to tell about sexual intercourse:

'It's a big thing. I don't think children's minds are
capable - it's a shame they should have to cope - let
them enjoy themselves at this age.'

Some class differences emerged both in flexibility of
approach and timing when parents were asked how old
children should be when they are first told where babies
come from. Middle-class parents were more likely to say
that a flexible approach should be adopted to the age of
telling about babies, but not about sexual intercourse
(43% compared with 29% of working-class parents for
telling about babies). One explanation for this is that
since middle-class parents are more in favour of the
first telling about where babies come from being done by
parents, they feel they have greater control over when
they should do the telling. It is also possible that
middle-class parents felt more in control of the
interview situation, and that working-class parents
answered more in terms of what was apparently expected.

When ages were given, middle-class parents suggested
younger ages for first telling about babies (a mean age
of 9.6 years compared with 10.6 years suggested by
working-class parents) but not for first telling about
sexual intercourse. This is in line with the differences reported by the young people (see Chapter 4).
The process also seems to be influenced by the sex of
the child. The data in Table 33 suggest that parents
think that children of their own sex should be told
earlier than children of the opposite sex. However,
differences in suggested ages for boys and girls
disappear when an appropriate age for first telling
about sexual intercourse is given.

TABLE 33   Mean ages suggested by parents for girls and
boys to learn about reproduction and sexual intercourse
from all sources

| | Where babies come from | | Sexual intercourse | |
	Mothers	Fathers	Mothers	Fathers
	Years	Years	Years	Years
Females	9.2 (53)	11.0 (44)	12.2 (53)	12.3 (53)
Males	10.5 (53)	10.1 (60)	12.3 (64)	12.0 (61)
All	9.9(106)	10.5(104)	12.2(117)	12.1(114)

( )   Numbers in brackets represent base number, which is
      less than number asked the question since some did
      not mention an age in their reply.

PARENTS' ACTIONS OR OMISSIONS

Although nearly all the parents interviewed felt that
ideally one or both parents should be involved in talking
to children at some stage about reproduction (90%) and
sexual intercourse (79%), when they were asked if they
had ever discussed these subjects with their own child,
far fewer said that they had (they were asked, 'Have you
ever talked to _____ about where babies come from? And
about sexual intercourse?'). Less than half of them
remembered ever discussing where babies come from, and
just over a quarter said they had ever discussed sexual
intercourse. Table 34 shows that more mothers said they
had talked to their daughters about babies than did
fathers, and more fathers had talked to sons, as they had
said was appropriate. More fathers said they had
discussed both subjects with boys than fathers asked
about girls. Also more mothers said they had discussed
babies with boys than fathers said they had with girls.
     Looking at the proportion of parents who said they had
initiated the talks they had had with their own child,
the data suggest that fathers play a less active role
than mothers. More of the fathers said that the
discussions about babies had been initiated by their son
or daughter (61% compared with 25%). Although the numbers
of parents who commented on the question of how they felt
at the time of the discussion are small (99 mothers and
60 fathers commented on discussions about babies, and 56
mothers and 37 fathers commented about sexual intercourse),
the following comments give an indication of how some of

TABLE 34 Proportions of mothers and fathers who believed they should tell about reproduction at some stage and those who had talked about it

	Mothers asked about boys	Mothers asked about girls	Fathers asked about boys	Fathers asked about girls
	%	%	%	%
Said mothers/fathers should ever tell about babies	57	91	69	27
Said they had talked about babies	46	66	55	22
Said mothers/fathers should ever tell about sexual intercourse	36	81	62	22
Said they had talked about sexual intercourse	25	39	30	16
Number of mothers/fathers (= 100%)	91	95	89	74

them reacted. The majority of mothers (62%) and fathers
(57%) said that they had felt no particular emotion:
    'Just the sort of things that kids ask and you tell
    them, there's no point in hiding it.'
Some (11% of mothers and 13% of fathers) admitted to
feeling embarrassed):
    'Embarrassment, but we realised he ought to know.'
A few (9%) of mothers and 3% of fathers) expressed
pleasure:
    'I was pleased that we'd seen it [a film] together
    and that we'd discussed it. I told her more about
    it.'
A small number of fathers (8%) said they had been shocked
or surprised when they had been asked to talk about where
babies come from, and this increased to 11% when they
commented on the way they had felt at the time they
discussed sexual intercourse. On this subject, more
fathers said they had felt embarrassed (22%) and fewer
mothers (5%); but mothers also expressed concern with
the way they were doing the telling (21%) - concern that
they might not be doing the telling properly:
    'Anxious primarily because I had to know that he knew.'
Amongst those parents who had talked about reproduction
were a small group (20) who said that they did not think
parents should tell their children. They represent a
seventh (15%) of all those parents who had initially felt
that they should not be involved. The majority of them
were mothers (16) and they had mainly discussed the
subject in response to questions or comments from their
children. One mother who had done this said:
    'I don't think they need telling. We didn't tell
    ours, but they knew in plenty of time. I think it's
    human nature isn't it? Like the swallows flying back
    to Africa - they certainly know the way.'
She had reluctantly discussed the subject with her son,
when he was 17, because he asked questions about a newspaper article he had read.
    Middle-class parents were more likely to say they had
talked about sex at ages nearer to the ones they had
suggested as the best age to learn. The mean age at
which they said they had told their children about babies
was 9.0 years compared with 9.7 years for working-class
parents. Talking about sexual intercourse was recalled
as having happened at a later age, 13.2 years by middle-
class parents and 12.9 years for working-class parents.
    The main reasons given by those parents who had failed
to carry out their beliefs were that they thought their
children had already learned about reproduction at school
(17%):

'...she can think things out for herself and the school can fill in...books at school and in the library have always been available for her.'
Or from the other parent (13%):
'Her mother discussed it with her. I think it's better for the mother, and my wife is very capable and can put it in a decent way.'
Or had in some way discovered for themselves (18%):
'I just assumed he knows. I don't think I need to - he's reasonably level-headed and he knows my views.'
Other reasons included nervousness and embarrassment (5%), and the fact that their child had never raised the subject:
'She's never broached the subject and neither have I. It wasn't a taboo subject. It's like billiards - we haven't talked about that either.'

THE BEST WAY TO LEARN

We have already seen that most of these parents felt that they should be involved in some way in telling or talking to their children about sex. But learning is more than one person giving certain kinds of information to another, and so the parents were asked for their views on the best way for young people to learn about sex (they were asked: 'What do you think is the best way for boys/girls to learn about reproduction - I mean where babies come from and sexual intercourse?', and some parents mentioned more than one source in their answer). Just over half (51%) gave replies which centred on lessons at school. As one mother said:
'The best way is scientifically, through animals and so on - through their education. My son learned this way, as far as I know.'
Just over a third (36%) said that they thought it was best if young people learned at home from their parents, and one in four of these parents suggested that the information should be given by the parent of the same sex as the child. One mother said about girls:
'From their mothers first, then probably from their husbands - they'll get to know soon enough.'
Some parents described the best way as a combination of parent and teacher:
'It should be explained verbally by parents at first, then through lessons at school.'
Others (27%) recommended books or films:
'Give them a book, so long as they can read.'
'I suppose a good book might be as good as anything.'

A few parents (7%) felt that observation of pets and
animals was the best way:
> 'Roy always kept rabbits and things and I think it's
> always in their minds, even before they're old enough
> to know anything.'

Although when they were asked who should tell young
people nearly all the parents (90%) said that parents
should be involved in telling their children about sex,
far fewer of them felt that parental telling was the best
way to learn (36%). Add to this the information that less
than half of them had ever discussed babies or sex with
their own children, and we can see the extent of parental
ambivalence on the subject. Explanations for this have
already been offered, and include the reluctance of
parents to present their own sexuality to their children,
incest-taboos, embarrassment and uncertainty about their
ability to give information in the 'right' way. Certainly
parents and young people in this study were aware that
embarrassment between parents and children might inhibit
this form of learning:
> 'the best way to learn is from school - if we told
> them it could be a bit embarrassing; at school it's a
> lesson and that's that.'

Similar feelings were expressed by a young person:
> 'Well, I suppose it's a good idea to have someone
> parents can trust giving sex education lessons, as
> some of the parents could be embarrassed.'

It is possible that in addition to finding it difficult
to raise the subject, some parents feel they are not as
well equipped to deal with the subject as others; 88% of
these mothers and fathers said that they thought their son
or daughter was better informed about these things than
they were at the same age (the parents were asked: 'Do
you think _____ knows more, less or about the same as you
did when you were his/her age about sex and birth
control?'). However, more parents had talked to their
children about sex than thought it was the best way to
learn. Reasons for this include the fact that children
initiated discussions and parents felt they should answer
their questions, possibly because they realised that the
schools were not fulfilling their role, and because films
and books on the subject are not readily available.

BELIEFS AND ACTIONS ABOUT BIRTH CONTROL

Compared with telling about reproduction, fewer parents
felt that one or both parents should be the first ones to
tell their children about birth control (41% compared with

71%), and there is a strong indication that some of them
felt it was best done outside the family altogether.
When they were asked what they thought was the best way
for boys or girls to learn about contraception, a third
(32%), mentioned parents alone or in conjunction with
another source; just over a third mentioned teachers and
lessons at school, and 31% mentioned medical personnel
and discussion 'with someone who knows':

> 'The doctor. I draw a distinction here between parents
> and qualified people. To me intercourse is a natural
> thing and one can speak naturally about it. But birth
> control is an interference with a natural thing and
> therefore it would be easier for a doctor to deal with
> it more sensitively. And the doctor would have an
> expert knowledge as distinct from the half-knowledge
> that a parent would have.'

Over a quarter (28%) thought that books and films should
be used in this context, either on their own or as aids
to discussion:

> 'It depends whether they are that way inclined or not.
> Obviously if they want to use it, if they want to have
> sex, then they should go to the family planning. But
> if they just want to know about it they could just have
> a book or have a discussion about it.'

A few parents thought they should learn through
experience or find out for themselves when they were
ready (3%):

> 'When they're capable of knowing what sexual inter-
> course is and what its effects are, and by then they
> should have a sufficiently enquiring mind to find out.'

A third of these parents thought parents telling was
the best way to learn about birth control, but nearly
two-thirds of them thought parents should talk to their
children about it at some stage. Mothers and fathers
agreed that it was inappropriate for fathers alone to
tell daughters and equal proportions of mothers and
fathers thought that mothers should tell daughters and
that fathers should tell sons. Their views diverged on
joint telling of boys, when it appeared that more fathers
than mothers (44% compared with 25%) saw this as the
relevant telling situation and 3% of fathers thought
mothers alone should tell boys, but 8% of mothers thought
they should. Once again, parents seem to agree on their
roles in relation to girls, but not in relation to boys.

There were no class differences between parents who
gave some information and those who did not. In more than
half of the instances (55%) the parents said they had been
the ones to raise the subject. Where the parents reported
that the young people had raised the subject they were

more likely to say that a daughter rather than a son had
initiated discussion (30% of parents said daughters had
raised the subject compared with 15% of parents recalling
sons raising the issue). The reported mean age of parent-
child discussions was 14.9 years, later than the 'ideal'
age for talking about birth control suggested by the
parents (13.4 years).

In conclusion, of the four topics parents were asked
about, birth control was the one least often discussed
(27% had discussed birth control). Mothers were more
likely to have discussed it, and they told girls more
often than boys. It seems likely from the comments made
in relation to birth control that they felt less confident
about discussing this subject. They also gave the
impression that, by talking about birth control, they
might 'encourage' their daughters to have sex:

'I don't believe in all this pill at 16 - put it this
way, if you've got an 'H' bomb you've got a deterrent -
I think the pill is not a deterrent, it encourages
them.'

BELIEFS AND ACTIONS IN RELATION TO VENEREAL DISEASE

In contrast to birth control, venereal disease was a topic
which most parents approached with enthusiasm. Many of
the interviewers commented that this was a subject which
inspired a keen response in the parents being interviewed.
Nearly all of them thought that young people should be
told about venereal disease (97%), but fewer of them
thought that one or both parents should be involved in
the telling (33%). More parents thought that teachers
should assume a role here, since 44% suggested that a
teacher should provide this information either alone or
as well as a parent. More mothers than fathers (41%
compared with 25%) thought that children should learn from
parents, but they were no more likely to say that the
telling should be done by both parents.

As on the subject of birth control, mothers and fathers
were in agreement that fathers alone should not tell
daughters about venereal disease, and fathers also felt
that mothers should not do the telling alone with boys.
On this subject the same disagreement between parents
arose in relation to boys as in telling about birth
control, since 8% of mothers asked about boys thought they
alone should be the ones to tell them. Middle-class
mothers were more likely to recommend that both parents
should tell their children about venereal disease than
working-class mothers (45% compared with 22%).

In actions, too, parents were more likely to say they
had talked about venereal disease than they were to say
they had talked about birth control (35% said they had
done so compared with 27% who had talked about birth
control). Mothers remained the ones most likely to say
they had done the talking (42% compared with 28% of
fathers) but daughters were as likely to have been told
as sons. The mean age at which these parents said they
had told their children suggests that they talk about
venereal disease at about the same age as they talk about
birth control (14.8 years).

There is little doubt from the comments parents made
about what young people should be told about venereal
disease, that they saw it as a sanction against permissiveness and promisuity. Two-thirds of these comments could
be categorised as containing warnings:

'that it can ruin their lives and will stop them having
a happy married life if they catch VD when they're
young.'
'How it's caused, what causes it by going out with
dirty people. That it can be damaging to them.'
'Show them a few photographs, especially of people who
haven't been treated, tell them about the mental
aspect.'

They should be:

'frightened by the thought of babies deformed at
birth. She saw it at Madame Tussaud's in Blackpool.
I think it frightened her.'

In a way, more insight into parental attitudes to sex is
gained from their attitudes to and comments about venereal
disease than from any of the other topics. The fulfilment
of sexual relationships and pleasure involved were rarely
mentioned anywhere, but the vigour with which they
commented on venereal disease suggests that Victorian
morality still abounds. As Gagnon and Simon point out,
'society is really closer to eliminating syphilis than it
is prepared to admit, and the epidemic of gonorrhoea is
as much a consequence of misplaced medical priorities as
it is of promiscuity' (1973, p.113). There are few signs
from these parents of what Gagnon and Simon have described
as 'the growing belief that sex is a potentially positive,
joyous, and enriching experience that no longer is the
sole possession of an alienated and radical minority in
society'.

PARENTS' VIEWS OF PREMARITAL SEX

The parents interviewed were more likely than their

children to say that they disapproved of sex before
marriage. A third (33%) of these mothers and fathers said
outright that they disapproved, with a further 16% saying
they had mixed feelings with a leaning towards disapproval.
Some of their spontaneous comments revealed the extent of
this disapproval:

'I'm 100% anti - if you behave like rabbits before
then you will behave like rabbits after. No person
will remain faithful if they indulge beforehand.'

Some were repressive:

'One shouldn't allow people to fornicate willy-nilly
without some deterrent being placed upon them.'

On the other hand, one in four parents (26%) said they
approved or were inclined to approve:

'Something I've never worried about - doesn't bother
me - I know Andrew and his girlfriend sleep together.
I think it is good to get to know each other, it's all
part of a relationship.'

Twenty-two per cent said they had mixed feelings about it:

'I would say it is not right, but in these times, I
don't know. I think it's all wrong, but my lot keep
telling me, in a few years there won't be any such
thing as marriage.'

Table 35 shows the differences in attitudes between
parents and young people.

Although there are wide differences between parents
and young people's attitudes, they follow the same
patterns: boys more likely to 'approve' than girls,
fathers more likely to 'approve' than mothers. The
parental social class differences reveal the same tendency
for more of the working-class groups to say they 'approve'
of sex before marriage (8% of middle-class mothers said
they approved compared with 12% of working-class mothers;
16% of middle-class fathers compared with 32% of working-
class fathers).

One of the most interesting, if not unexpected,
findings was that mothers who were being interviewed about
their daughters were more likely to say they disapproved
of sex before marriage (63%), compared with 47% of mothers
asked about their sons. This mother said it for them all:

'Very difficult. It depends on sex. But then for a
girl - more important for a girl to protect her
virginity than for a man.'

American evidence suggests (Reiss, 1970) that as a
group married people are twice as likely to disagree with
premarital sex as unmarried people, and that parents with
older children are most likely to disagree with it. This
is explained in terms of responsibility for their children,
which would also explain the higher degree of disapproval

TABLE 35 Parents' and young people's attitudes to premarital sex

	Males	Females	All teenagers	Mothers	Fathers	All parents
	%	%	%	%	%	%
Approved	60	37	49	12	24	18
Mixed feelings						
More to approve	13	14	13	8	7	8
Equal	15	28	21	24	20	22
More to disapprove	4	10	7	18	15	16
Disapproved	7	10	9	36	29	33
Other comment/don't know/can't say	1	1	1	2	5	3
Number = 100%	779*	771*	1,550	186	163	349

* 3 excluded because inadequate.

from mothers with daughters. Our evidence certainly backs
this up, although the figure Reiss quotes for the proportion of 'disapproving' adults in the American population
in 1967 is much higher than the proportion of our parents
expressing disapproval (77% compared with 33% outright
disapproval; 77% compared with 49% if mixed feelings
towards disapproval are included).

SUMMARY

Parents feel that they ought to be involved in telling
their children about reproduction and sex. Mothers assume
a greater responsibility than fathers for this, especially
in the early stages of the process - telling where babies
come from. Fathers support this both verbally and by
allowing mothers to 'do' most of the informing.

Mothers are concerned that children, especially
daughters, should not learn about sex too soon.

Many parents say that the best way for young people to
learn about sex is through lessons at school.

A minority of parents remembered having had discussions
about sex with their children. Mothers and their
daughters had talked most. Parents agreed that fathers
should only talk to girls if it were a joint parental
discussion.

The gap between parental beliefs and intentions was
greatest for the subject of birth control. Mothers were
more likely to have discussed it with daughters, but many
parents indicated that they felt less capable of giving
information about this subject, and recommended teachers,
doctors and books as alternative sources.

Parents were strongly in favour of young people being
told about venereal disease, and more of them had discussed
it with their own children than had discussed birth control.
Their attitudes to what information should be given reveal
strong inclinations to use the 'horrors' of venereal
disease as a sanction against permissiveness and
promiscuity.

7

FAMILY RELATIONSHIPS

Sexuality has only recently become part of the literature
of sociology and suffers, as Plummer points out in his
book 'Sexual Stigma' (1975), from the lack of a theoretical base. He describes how past attempts to explain
sexual behaviour have been dominated by psychological
theories maintaining that sexual drive is a physiological
factor which individuals 'learn' to control. Attempts
to understand sexuality have been mainly descriptive
(Kinsey, Schofield, etc.), until 1973, when Gagnon and
Simon published their interactionist study 'Sexual
Conduct'. The discussion now centres on whether sexuality
is the result of basic instinctual biological forces
struggling to get out and being controlled by social
forces, or whether it is initially shaped by the social
meanings attributed to it. The interactionist position
as stated by its proponents (Plummer; Gagnon and Simon)
is that sexuality has no meaning other than that given
to it in social situations. At the same time it does not
deny that biological and psychological processes are
involved in sexuality - as Plummer puts it: 'The
sociological task requires that the sociologist demonstrates the social nature of sexuality while remaining
sensitive to the boundaries imposed by biology and
psychology.'
    It was suggested at the beginning of this study that
there were three main sources of learning about sex:
parents, friends and the formal educational process. The
data indicate that if young people had been told about
human reproduction by one or both of their parents, they
were more likely to say they had learned at an earlier
age (9.5 years compared with 11 years).
    Another important finding was that over half the young
people did not learn (or did not remember learning) about
sexual intercourse at the same time as they learned about

reproduction but at a later age. The parents interviewed also indicated that they were less likely to talk about sexual intercourse to their children and if they did, it was talked about at a later age.

This separation in learning of the act of intercourse from the reproductive functions of the body has significance in terms of the way meanings are given to sexuality by parents (and others). If, as Gagnon and Simon suggest, sexual meanings are first created in the family situation through the processes of negative labelling and non-labelling (i.e., parents respond to the child's imputed sexual activity by saying 'don't do that', and also with responses that are ambiguous and ill-defined), when the adolescent looks back to the way in which he was told (if he was told by his parents) he will impute or perceive that his mother or father was reluctant to tell him about the act of intercourse, since to separate the act from the process of reproduction is to distort the true process. What kind of meaning does the adolescent give to his parents' views of sexuality (and therefore in part to his own) when he realises that they have initially suppressed or ignored telling him about the most intimate part of the process? As Gagnon and Simon say: 'Learning about sex in our society is learning about guilt; conversely, learning how to manage sexuality constitutes learning how to manage guilt.' How much more accurate is this for the children who could not remember their parents ever telling them about sex at all (60% of the boys in this study and 36% of the girls)? From the position of knowledge, the adolescent might look back and ask himself why his parents did not give him the information which he considers it necessary to have.

Our data suggest that working-class boys are more likely to be sexually experienced than other boys and the girls of both groups. They also suggest that they are less likely to use effective contraception. It seems likely, therefore, that their attitudes to sex are different. Attempts to explain why this is so are surrounded by difficulties. This study is particularly limited in this respect because it captured attitudes and behaviour at a single point in time. However, current relationships with parents may well reflect the past, and so they are examined here in an attempt to explain behaviour patterns.

We know from our findings that working-class parents as a whole were less likely to say they disapproved of sex before marriage (43% compared with 58% of middle-class parents), particularly where their sons were concerned (33% of working-class fathers asked about sons said they disapproved of sex before marriage compared with 44% of middle-class fathers; 43% of working-class mothers asked about sons said they disapproved of sex before marriage compared with 53% of middle-class mothers). It is possible that this 'lesser' degree of disapproval is communicated to the boys and that they feel freer to become sexually experienced. It is also possible that they feel less inclined to take notice of their parents' attitudes.

When the parent-young people relationships are examined, differences emerge which suggest a possible link between 'ease' of communication and sexual behaviour. Relationships are, of course, extremely difficult to quantify, and there must be reservations about these kinds of data. However, one measure used was to ask the young people how easy or difficult they found it to talk to their mothers and fathers about things that were important to them. There were no differences between boys and girls in the study as a whole (61% of boys said they found it easy to talk to their mothers compared with 63% of the girls). But when the groups are analysed in terms of sex, class and sexual experience, differences emerge which suggest that parent-teenage relationships might be affected by teenage sexual behaviour (or alternatively, that the relationship influences their sexual activity).

Being sexually experienced did not make any difference to how easy working-class boys found it to talk to their mothers, and it seemed that possibly fewer working-class boys who were not sexually experienced found it easy to talk to their fathers. Since the data on parental attitudes to sex before marriage suggest that working-class mothers and fathers are less likely to disapprove of this activity, it is possible that sexual experience makes no difference to the ease with which they talk to their mothers and is an indication that relationships do not suffer because of it, or alternatively that they encourage it. On the other hand, sexually experienced middle-class boys are less likely to say that they found it easy to talk to their mothers than middle-class boys who were not sexually experienced, a possible indication that they felt their communication with their mothers to be restricted by their sexual experience. Sexually experienced working-class girls were also less likely to say they found it easy to talk to their mothers about things that were important to them, which could also be an indication that they 'felt' their mothers' disapproval. All the sexually experienced young people were asked if their parents knew they were sexually experienced, and although there were differences between boys and girls,

TABLE 36 Proportion of young people who said they found it easy to talk to their parents about things which were important to them

	Middle class	Working class	All***
Boys about fathers			
Sexually experienced boys	43% (152)	45% (258)	46% (409)
Non-sexually experienced boys	44% (148)	39% (157)	43% (304)
All boys**	43% (310)	42% (431)	44% (740)
Boys about mothers			
Sexually experienced boys	54% (152)	60% (258)	59% (422)
Non-sexually experienced boys	70% (148)	58% (157)	65% (314)
All boys**	61% (310)	59% (431)	61% (762)
Girls about fathers			
Sexually experienced girls	30% (137)	24% (194)	27% (323)
Non-sexually experienced girls	40% (136)	28% (212)	34% (356)
All girls**	35% (289)	26% (427)	31% (718)
Girls about mothers			
Sexually experienced girls	57% (137)	56% (194)	58% (349)
Non-sexually experienced girls	63% (136)	*70% (212)	69% (367)
All girls**	60% (289)	64% (427)	63% (756)

( ) Figures in brackets are the numbers on which the percentages are based (= 100%).

* Difference is significant at 5% level.

** Including those young people who refused to say whether they were sexually experienced.

*** Including those young people whose fathers' occupations were unclassified or armed forces but excluding young people with no father or no mother.

there were no class differences in the proportions who
said they did. Forty-four per cent of middle-class and
working-class boys said their mothers knew; 39% of middle-
class girls and 35% of working-class girls. Slightly
fewer working-class boys reported that their mothers had
expressed anger or disapproval on finding out or being
told (5% compared with 9% of middle-class boys and
working-class girls, and 12% of middle-class girls).
Although this evidence is by no means conclusive, it is
reinforced a little when we look at the topics the young
people mentioned when they were asked if there was anything they would never talk to their mothers and fathers
about. Of those who said there were things they would
never discuss with their mother (41% of young people),
three out of four mentioned sex, and personal relationships with a member of the opposite sex. The comparable
proportion for fathers was two out of three. Sexually
experienced girls were more likely to mention this as a
topic they would never discuss with their mothers than
girls who were not sexually experienced (32% compared
with 18%). Although boys were equally reluctant to
discuss sex with their mothers, being sexually experienced
did not influence whether they mentioned the subject or
not (32% of sexually experienced boys compared with 27%
of those who were not sexually experienced). One girl
explained it as natural reluctance:
    'Yes, personal things with boyfriends - but I haven't
    kept anything from her yet - I haven't felt the need
    to yet, I haven't reached the stage yet. But I
    wouldn't tell her if I had intercourse. No girl would
    tell her mother.'
One boy attributed his reluctance to embarrassment:
    'Yes, sex. Not because I didn't want to but because
    I think it would embarrass her.'
And another boy described feelings whenever sex was
mentioned:
    'Yes, sex. She just seems to shut up and think "he
    knows and that's that". She's a bit shy over these
    things, and my dad is. They think "he knows it" but
    wouldn't talk to you about it.'
The implications of these kinds of comments - that
young people feel they cannot discuss sex with their
parents because of embarrassment or because they are
expected to know and not talk about it, or because their
parents would disapprove - indicate that there is some
truth in the explanation that sexuality is given meaning
by social situations.
    Another clearer indication that sexual experience
affects relationships with parents is suggested by the

findings on whom the young people named as being the most
important influence for them. Table 37 shows that for
all social class groups, young people who were sexually
experienced were less likely to name their parents.

TABLE 37   Proportions of young people saying one or both
parents had been the most important influence on the way
they thought and acted by sexual experience and social
class

	Sexually experienced	Not sexually experienced
Middle-class males	53% (152)	65% (147)
Working-class males	47% (258)	60% (157)
All males*	49% (433)	61% (322)
Middle-class females	51% (137)	65% (137)
Working-class females	42% (194)	63% (212)
All females*	45% (357)	63% (377)

*   Including 41 boys and 54 girls whose fathers'
    occupations were armed forces or unclassified.
( )Base numbers are in brackets after percentages.

This relationship between sexual experience and the
stated influence of parents is complicated by other
variables like age, sex and social class. As children
grow older they are obviously more likely to find other
people whom they regard as influential and they are more
likely to become sexually experienced. We also know that
girls are less likely to become sexually experienced at
as early an age as boys. The class differences in child-
rearing patterns observed by researchers like the Newsons
and Douglas, and in methods of communication established
by Bernstein, might lead us to expect differences in
adolescent sexual behaviour. Differences of the kind
observed in this study have also been found in other
studies, but there is no clearly established empirical
explanation for it - as this extract from 'Sexual Conduct'
(Gagnon and Simon, 1973, p.44) illustrates:
    Social class differences also appear to be significant,
    although both in the work of Kinsey and that of Kagan
    and Moss, they appear as more important factors for
    males than for females. Some part of this is due to
    aspects of sex-role learning which vary by social
    class. Differences in the legitimacy of expressing
    aggression or perhaps merely differences in modes of
    expressing aggression come immediately to mind. Another

difference is the degree to which sex-role models
display a capacity for *heterosociality*. The
frequently noted pattern of the sexual segregation of
social life among working-class and lower-class populations may make the structuring of later sexual activity,
particularly during adolescence, actually less complicated.

Given the acknowledge complexity of relationships between
sexual activity and sex, age and social class, and also
the limitations of our data, it is not possible to
establish a direct causal relationship between family
relationships and sexual experience. What is demonstrated
by the data presented here is that for some groups
becoming sexually experienced affects communication between
parent and child or vice-versa, and for all social class
groups sexual experience lessens the importance of parental
influence. In this respect the view that parents are
necessarily an appropriate source of information and advice
on sexual matters or birth control during adolescence
needs to be reconsidered.

This is reinforced when parental involvement in
discussions about sex is analysed. Although data presented
earlier suggest that middle-class teenagers were more
likely to say they had learned about sex from their
parents, there is no evidence to suggest that these
differences relate to sexual behaviour. Working-class
boys were still more likely to be sexually experienced
than other groups when the factor of first being told
about sex by parents is introduced. It is not surprising
that there is no direct link between learning about sex
from parents and sexual behaviour, since learning is part
of a total cultural pattern. Also, learning is a process
and it is not possible to incorporate all the parts of
the process into quantifiable data. Partly to offset
this, the next section presents data from 614 parallel
interviews with family members. As explained in the
introduction, interviews were conducted at a random 1 in
4 addresses with young people and one of their parents.
Of the 614 'family' members interviewed, 167 were mothers
and 140 were fathers. Their sons were interviewed in 150
cases and their daughters in 157. Table 38 shows the
proportions of mothers and fathers who were asked questions
about sons and daughters. The difference between the
number of mother-daughter pairs and the number of father-
daughter pairs was not statistically significant and the
characteristics of the young people in this group were
similar to those of all the young people interviewed in
respect of sex, age and marital status.

TABLE 38   Relationship of the family members interviewed

	%
Mothers and sons	25
Mothers and daughters	29
Fathers and sons	24
Fathers and daughters	22
Number of parent/young people pairs (= 100%)	307

Before these findings are presented some discussion of
their validity is necessary. There were two reasons for
interviewing parents as part of this study. One was to
gather their collective attitudes to sex education and to
see how they themselves told their own children about sex
and birth control. The other was to be able, by interviewing members of the same family, to look in greater
detail at their accounts of the process and the similarity
or otherwise of their experiences and attitudes. In a
way these parallel interviews made it possible to check
the accuracy of our findings. But the most important
aspect of this part of the study lies in the agreement
observed between parent and child, and not in a discussion
of the discrepant accounts. If two people give similar
accounts of events independently, it is more likely that
these accounts are accurate. As Niemi points out in his
study 'How Family Members Perceive Each Other' (1974):
   Neither the students' nor the parents' reports can be
   considered a standard by which to judge the accuracy
   of the others' perceptions. It is entirely possible
   that both students' and parents' reports do not
   accurately reflect the true family situation....
   Technically, then, we cannot determine here whether
   students' or parents' reports are accurate pictures
   of family life. Nevertheless, if considerable
   student-parent agreement is found, it would strengthen
   the view that respondents do give reasonably accurate
   reports of family living. (p.102)
He previously described other problems of working with
family data:
   The validity of family-level data has been questioned
   most frequently and most seriously with regard to
   reports of family structure and relationships among
   family members. It has been charged that both
   children and parents...bias their responses to make
   themselves and their families appear more socially

acceptable. Moreover, it has been suggested that
different members of a family often present varying
accounts of the same phenomenon, so that the descriptions of any single member cannot be relief upon. (p.6)
These problems of perception have been commented on
earlier and are, in our case, compounded by memory and
the passage of time. Discrepant accounts of whether or
how a young person was told about reproduction, sexual
intercourse and birth control by his parents do not
necessarily mean that one of the two accounts is false.
Similar reports are, however, an indication that the
accounts are likely to be reasonably accurate. Given
these reservations, we compare now the young people and
parent accounts of sex education in the family, then the
similarity or otherwise of their attitudes to sex before
marriage and abortion, and finally their relationships
with each other.

TALKING TO EACH OTHER ABOUT REPRODUCTION

Over half (54%) of the parents and young people gave the
same account of whether or not they had discussed where
babies come from during childhood or adolescence. A third
of the accounts (33%) were discrepant. Where there were
discrepancies fewer parents reported having talked about
reproduction than young people reported parents having
told them (11% compared with 22%). If there is a bias
towards 'socially acceptable' answers, it would appear
that the young people are more likely to do this than
parents, assuming that parents telling about reproduction
is considered the acceptable answer. Table 39 shows the
proportions of parents and young people who gave similar
accounts of learning about babies, sexual intercourse and
birth control within the family.
    Although the characteristics of each group inevitably
reflected those established from the larger sample because
this group is part of that sample, it seems worth
repeating that boys were more likely to be found in
category 2, thus reflecting the finding that boys are
less likely to be told about sexual matters by their
parents than girls. The only other category in which sex
differences occurred was in the discrepant accounts of
birth control discussions. Here girls were more likely
to say that they had not talked to their parents about
birth control when their parents reported the opposite.
Explanations for this cannot be substantiated but possibly
arose from differing perceptions of what constituted
'talking about birth control'. When the parents were asked

TABLE 39   Parent/young people reports of discussions about
reproduction, sexual intercourse and birth control

	Where babies come from	Sexual inter-course	Birth control
	%	%	%
1 Both said subject discussed	24	10	16
2 Both said subject not discussed	30	52	43
3 Discrepant accounts	33	29	32
4 Either said 'don't know'	13	9	9
Number of parent/young people pairs (= 100%)	307	307	307

what aspects of birth control methods they had discussed
with their child a third (30%) of those who had talked
about the subject said they had only talked 'in generali-
ties' or 'vaguely' about birth control. These kinds of
discussions could easily be discounted as irrelevant or
forgotten.

Although there were no social class differences between
the groups, the parents whose reports were similar to
their children's, in the sense that both parties said they
had talked about the subjects, were more likely to have
educational qualifications than those parents who said the
subject had not been discussed (50% compared with 24%).

The most important implication of these findings,
however, is that where parents and young people said that
discussions about reproduction and birth control had taken
place, those discussions had been of such a kind that both
sides remembered them. This could mean that embarrassment
was so strong on these occasions that they took on a
'never-to-be-forgotten' character. But another finding
suggests that this is not the case. Where similar reports
were given by parent and young person that the subject had
been discussed, the teenagers were more likely to say that
they were very satisfied with the way they had learned.
This too could be said to be simply a reflection of the
findings from the wider sample, but it does also suggest
that the quality of the discussions within these families
was such that it enabled the young people to feel satis-

TABLE 40   Similarity of reports of talking about sexual
intercourse by young people's satisfaction with the way
they learned about sex

| Young people's satisfaction | Similar accounts | | Discrepant accounts |
	Subject discussed	Subject not discussed	
	%	%	%
Very satisfied	47	16	30
Satisfied	7	28	29
Dissatisfied	46	56	41
Number of parent/ young people pairs (= 100%)	30	161	90

fied with the way they had learned about sex.   The excerpt
which follows illustrates what happened in one family
where both parent and young person gave similar accounts
about their discussions and where the young person said
she was very satisfied with the way she had learned about
sex:
    Felicity was the eldest girl in a middle-class family.
    She had first learned where babies come from when she
    was seven and her mother was pregnant.   'My mother was
    expecting my brother.   I wasn't told everything at
    once.   The initiative from the beginning was left to
    me so that they'd know what stage of thinking I was
    at, and when I was around ten or eleven the questions
    I asked tended to get deeper and deeper so that a full
    explanation was necessary.'   She said she had been told
    about sexual intercourse by her mother and father and
    by a visiting marriage guidance counsellor at school.
    Her mother had told her about periods when she was 11,
    two years before she began to menstruate.   'I was glad
    that it was personal rather than being handed a book.
    My own view is that if you've got the right nature,
    that is not easily embarrassed, or you're close, to
    speak about something from personal experience is
    better than to have a book which is perhaps dry and
    impersonal.'
        A series of sex education lessons had been given in
    secondary school in her fourth year, which she thought
    was 'a bit late - but better late than never'.   A
    visiting speaker had talked about 'sexual behaviour and

the way your body works. Then as far as I can remember
we had three [lessons] on birth control. No guidance
at all morally.' 'I think the most beneficial of the
series was those concerned with birth control rather
than actually sexual behaviour because nine out of ten
knew about general sex education but comparatively few
knew about birth control.' No offers of opportunities
to discuss sex outside lessons had been made, but 'I
think there were some members of staff who would have
been happy to discuss it if you'd asked, but it was
never mentioned publicly as a service.'
     She said she had discussed the whole range of
sexual topics presented, except masturbation, with her
mother and father, with a male and female friend, but
said she could not single out one person who had been
most helpful because they had all been helpful in
different ways: 'Parents because they tell me the
facts of life if I asked them questions, and I still
ask their views. Friends tend to be more personal
problems, our own views - I feel that getting on for
half of good sex education is learned from each other -
the personal side anyway.' Her comments on the way
she had learned about sex were 'I can't honestly think
of any way it could have been improved. I can
certainly think of lots of ways it could have been
worse. I was told in very simple, straightforward
language, very matter of fact, which I think is what
a child needs.' On the best way to learn about sex
she said: 'To be told personally rather than handed a
book. Books are fine for supplementing what you've
already been told, but I don't think they can replace
the personal touch.' Her knowledge of all methods of
birth control was comprehensive and accurate. She
gave eight correct answers out of nine on the self-
administered questionnaire, with one 'don't know'.
She thought the birth control lessons at school had
been 'very informative and very necessary, I should
imagine, in just about every school'. She had
discussed birth control with her mother, father, male
and female friends and female relatives. She felt she
could not say who had been most helpful to talk to
about birth control: 'Because I've never gone with any
particular problems about birth control, it's just
come up in the conversation.' Her reactions to the
way she had learned about birth control were positive:
'I think that outside school, the time and the atmosphere are so often wrong. When it's part of the
curriculum and you have to sit and listen I think you
have to give it a proper hearing rather than waiting

till you had to or wanted to find out.' She felt she
knew enough about birth control 'for the moment anyway.
I don't know everything about birth control, but I
know enough for the moment anyway. I wouldn't refuse
the information if it came my way, but I don't feel
yet that I want to go out and seek more.' She thought
the best way to learn about birth control was 'to be
taught in school. But I also think you need more
books for this than for sexual intercourse because the
act of intercourse never will change ... whereas birth
control is essentially scientific and science is
constantly changing and improving, so I think you have
to keep up to date with what the latest developments
are.' She said she would prefer to go to a birth
control clinic for professional advice on birth control
'because unless you've got a medical problem and the
pill is making you ill, there's no point in going to
your doctor because he is essentially for ill people.
And because birth control clinics by their very nature
specialise in that and will therefore have all the up-
to-date information.' She said she found her own
doctor easy to talk to because 'for the majority of
the time he understands, he listens'. She also felt
that he had time to discuss things with her.

She said she was not sexually experienced and disapproved of sex before marriage for herself, but 'for
me it's wrong but I wouldn't say I disapproved of
anyone who did. Personally I'm against it. I couldn't
really understand why at first - that was when I
became a Christian. I started to take more notice of
what the Bible said and now through what the Bible has
to say and other things to do with life and living...
we come to the conclusion that it's right because I've
seen what happens when you break up and you've been
sleeping with your boyfriend - the tragedy it brings.
I think if you really love each other the chances are
you'll get married anyway, so you might as well wait.'

Her parents had been one of the most important
influences on her life 'in general character building
and security. And I would add, they were responsible
for introducing me to the Christian faith which is of
prime importance to me anyway.' Both her mother and
father she found eask to talk to because 'they listen
and then, more important, they tell me what they think,
whether I'm right or wrong, yet they never judge.'
She talked seriously to both of them about her relationships with 'friends of both sexes', and her ambitions
for her career and 'everyday things that are important
to me'.

Her father (who was also interviewed) also said they
had a close relationship: 'It's a long-standing
relationship, it's always been the case. This is not
to say that I expect to be told everything and that
she has her private problems, there probably are.
It's easy to talk to her in view of the relationship
we have - we talk a lot about young people and a lot
of our free time is taken up with youth work.' He
thought that mothers and fathers should be involved
in telling girls about reproduction and sexual intercourse, 'the best way is to learn from parents when
they ask - by explaining the reproductive preliminaries
and then go on to sexual intercourse as an act of
pleasure'. When asked if he had talked to his daughter
about babies and sexual intercourse, his account
corresponded with hers. He said that the subject had
arisen from 'her questioning' and that he had felt
'quite natural, I had anticipated the question, it was
no shock and I was grateful for the opportunity. I can
remember it quite well - she was very casual, natural,
certainly not shocked or surprised. She was confident
that the information I gave her was correct.' He said
that both he and his wife disapproved of sex before
marriage.

ATTITUDES TO SEX BEFORE MARRIAGE

Generational differences in attitudes to sex before
marriage were expected and found to be substantial. It
seems likely that although parents themselves may have
had sex before they were married, as they raised families
and became responsible for the lives of their children
they would be more likely to express disapproval of
premarital sex as a kind of protective instinct. Reiss's
study of American adults found this to be the case (Reiss,
1971, p.169). However, although there are generational
differences, similar trends within the groups of young
people and parents were found to exist (see Chapter 6).
In this section it is possible to look more closely at
attitudes within the family and to see what effects, if
any, parental attitudes had on children's attitudes and
behaviour. Not surprisingly, nearly two-thirds of the
parents and young people expressed opposing attitudes to
sex before marriage. The direction of their disagreement
was nearly always caused because parents expressed disapproval and their children said that they approved.
Amongst the other families 21% of parent and young people
pairs said they approved, 9% held the same disapproving

attitude, and 4% expressed the same attitude saying they
had mixed feelings about the question. When these
categories were analysed by sex and social class, working-
class boys were more likely to be found in the category of
those who approved of sex before marriage along with their
parents. Although this has been said before, it is worth
repeating now that we have found similar attitudes within
the same families. It could explain why working-class
boys are more likely to be sexually experienced. If they
have parents who express approval of sex before marriage,
there is a possibility that they feel less inhibited
about becoming sexually experienced. Although it is far
from certain that parental attitudes to sex before
marriage influence their children's behaviour, there is
some evidence to suggest that attitudes within families
are similar, in spite of the generational differences.
Those few parents who said they approved of sex before
marriage had children who were more likely to say they
approved than the children of parents who said they disapproved (74% compared with 61%). It is possible, of
course, that parents change their attitudes once they
know that their teenage children have become sexually
experienced. Parents were not asked if they knew whether
their child was sexually experienced, but the young
people were asked if their parents knew. The findings
here indicate that those young people who said that their
parents knew or suspected they had sexual experience were
less likely to have one parent who said he or she disapproved of sex before marriage.

It is not possible to say definitely that these
parents' attitudes changed once they knew their son or
daughter to be sexually experienced because they were not
asked for their views at any other stage. The findings
on the relationship of parental knowledge and attitudes
in respect of sex before marriage, plus the findings on
similar attitudes existing within families, suggest a
connection between parental attitudes and teenage sexual
attitudes. It should not be said that parents who say
they approve of sex before marriage actively encourage
their children to become sexually experienced, or that
those who disapprove actively discourage teenage sexual
activity. But the fact that nearly half (44%) of those
parents whose children were not sexually experienced
disapproved compared with 19% of those parents who knew
about their child's sexual activity is a comment on the
importance of intra-family attitudes. It may be that
once they know about their child's sexual experience
parents are less likely to say they disapprove. On the
other hand, it is also possible that their inclination to

TABLE 41 Parental knowledge of teenage sexual experience (young people's report) by parental attitudes to sex before marriage (parents' report)

Parents' attitude to sex before marriage	Parents who knew	Parents who did not know	Parents whose child not sexually experienced	All parents
	%	%	%	%
Approved	32	24	14	18
Mixed to approved	11	11	7	8
Mixed – equally balanced	25	7	19	23
Mixed to disapproved	13	27	16	17
Disapproved	19	31	44	34
Number of parents (= 100%)	63	45	166	337*

* Including 42 parents who were not part of the paired group and 21 whose children were unsure of their knowledge, but excluding 12 parents whose attitude to sex before marriage could not be categorised.

be less disapproving does, in some way, allow their children to feel less inhibited about early sexual experience. Reiss (1970) points out that parents often collude in their teenage children's sexual activity by allowing them to have access to the home when they are out or away: 'The most common place for coitus is in the girl's home or the boy's home' (p.80). Although we have no comparable data, it does seem likely that some parents convey tacit approval of sexual activity to their teenage sons, or at least do not make a point of expressing disapproval.

If these findings are looked at in conjunction with the evidence in the preceding chapter that mothers asked about daughters were more likely to say they disapproved of sex before marriage than when they were asked about sons, and than fathers were when asked about sons, it would seem that parental attitudes may be influenced by the possible outcome of their children's behaviour. Thus mothers with teenage daughters, who might be at risk of unhappiness or stigma from a premarital pregnancy, are more likely to say they disapprove, possibly in the hope that this will protect their children. The social class analysis also suggests that there are cultural traditions which influence attitudes with regard to sons.

ATTITUDES TO ABORTION

On the question of attitudes to abortion, just over half the parents and young people expressed attitudes which were at variance. Amongst those who expressed the same attitudes, 29% said that they disapproved, 14% said that they approved of abortion, and 3% said that they had mixed feelings about the question. Similar findings occurred here as on the question of sex before marriage, that young people whose parents approved were more likely to approve than those young people whose parents said they disapproved of abortion (39% compared with 22%). One interesting finding here was that similar attitudes did not seem to be based on teenage knowledge of parental attitudes. The young people were asked for their own views on abortion, and also asked to say whether they though their mothers and fathers approved or disapproved. For those 307 cases where a direct comparison was possible, over a third of the teenagers said that they did not know what their parents' attitudes were (40%), and a third (31%) attributed the wrong attitude (mostly (23%) due to young people attributing a disapproving attitude when parents said they approved or had mixed feelings). Only

TABLE 42 Parents' and young people's recommended course of action for an unmarried pregnant teenage girl

| Recommended course of action | Young people | | | Parents | | All parents |
| | Male | Female | All young people | Mothers | Fathers | |
	%	%	%	%	%	%
Girl should have illegitimate baby	39	54	47	59	45	53
Girl should have abortion	44	32	38	16	34	24
Other solutions	16	13	14	24	19	22
Uncertain	1	1	1	1	2	1
Number of young people/parents (= 100%)	150	157	307	167	140	307

one in five of the young people (21%) recorded an accurate attitude for their parents, with a further 8% saying their parents were inclined to approval or disapproval when the parents said they positively approved or disapproved.

The transmission of attitudes and the importance of sex roles is emphasised when the answers to a question about what action a teenage girl should take if she became pregnant are examined. Parents and teenagers were asked to say whether she should marry someone she would not be happy with, have an illegitimate baby, or have an abortion; 40% of the parents and teenagers recommended the same course of action, and 38% suggested different solutions. Table 42 shows the proportions of girls and mothers and fathers and sons recommending each course of action.

Mothers and daughters were more likely to say that she should have an illegitimate child than fathers and sons, who were more in favour of abortion. Abortion is a more pertinent question for women, and it is not surprising that over half of these mothers and girls thought that a pregnant girl should choose to have an illegitimate baby when only a third of the girls and a sixth of the mothers thought the preferred outcome should be abortion.

On the whole the proportions of family members expressing similar attitudes to premarital sex and abortion, and the characteristics of the groups of young people and parents who expressed the same attitudes, suggest that parental influence, particularly between the same sex pairs, does not disappear during adolescence, and in some cases may be said to play a part in teenage sexual behaviour.

FAMILY RELATIONSHIPS AND COMMUNICATION

The parents' and young people's replies to questions of whether they found it easy or difficult to talk to each other about things that were important to them, seem to indicate that the teenagers found talking to their mothers easier than talking to their fathers. Tables 43 and 44 show that both boys and girls found it easier to communicate with their mothers than with their fathers.

TABLE 43   Mothers' views on talking to young people, and young people's views on talking to mothers

	Mothers' views		Teenagers' views	
Found talking	Mothers asked about male child	Mothers asked about female child	Male	Female
	%	%	%	%
Easy	58	76	54	69
Difficult	13	6	24	15
Sometimes easy, sometimes difficult	17	15	17	12
Other comments	12	3	5	4
Number of mothers/ young people (= 100%)	77	90	148*	156*

* 2 males and 1 female excluded because no mothers.

TABLE 44   Fathers' views on talking to young people, and young people's views on talking to fathers

	Fathers' views		Teenagers' views	
Found talking	Fathers asked about male child	Fathers asked about female child	Male	Female
	%	%	%	%
Easy	52	63	33	33
Difficult	17	19	30	27
Sometimes easy, sometimes difficult	27	12	26	24
Other comments	4	6	11	16
Number of fathers/ young people (= 100%)	73	67	144*	150*

* 6 males and 7 females excluded because no father.

The reasons given by the young people for finding
fathers difficult to talk to were mainly related to the
fact that fathers were not around as much as mothers
(7% said this):
'I rarely talk to him about things, perhaps because
I don't see so much of him. He doesn't get in till
6.30 p.m. and doesn't have a proper weekend, he just
has Wednesdays.'
Also that the teenagers did not feel close or did not get
on with their father (15%). This was often related to
the fact that the young people and fathers had opposing
views about things, and that young people thought their
fathers were 'old-fashioned' or 'too rigid' (12%):
'Because today it's changed like in a lot of ways.
When I talk to him he thinks about what he did in his
days and he treats you like you should do what he did
in his days.'
All these things were said about mothers, too, but to
a lesser extent. Understanding and compatibility were
more frequently mentioned in relation to being able to
talk to mothers easily (by 34% and 21% of all the young
people respectively, compared with 17% and 12% who
mentioned these characteristics in relation to fathers).
Mothers and fathers mentioned similar difficulties they
had in communication with their teenage sons and
daughters, sometimes attributing these difficulties to
the generation gap (11%):
'They don't listen, they think they know it all these
days.'
Also to the reason that they and their children had
differing or opposing views on things (9%).
It seems clear, therefore, that in many cases mothers
are the people whom teenagers feel 'easy' with, and with
whom they discuss 'important' matters within the family.
The reasons why this was so varied from family to family,
but centred round maternal understanding and willingness
to listen:
'She's very understanding. Someone you can confide
in.'
'We think very much the same about - oh, just everything. She's very willing to listen to my views
and my friends', than even people of her own generation.'
'She's brought me up and learned me to talk to her.
She just learned me to speak freely to her.'
These findings would seem to indicate that more often
than not mothers take a greater share of the 'education'
of their children in sexual matters, and are more likely
to be involved in discussions about sex. More teenagers

feel 'easier' about talking to their mothers than to their fathers.

SUMMARY

Agreement between parent-teenage reports on discussions about reproduction, sexual intercourse and birth control within the family reflect the findings based on the young people reports, that boys are less likely to be told about these things by their parents, and that sexual intercourse is a subject infrequently discussed.

Where family reports do coincide and state that sex has been discussed, the young people were more likely to say they were satisfied with the way they had learned about sex.

In spite of wide generational differences in approval of sex before marriage, there is evidence that working-class parents of sons are less likely to say they disapprove, and that this in turn may make it easier for working-class boys to have sexual experience at an earlier age.

Attitudes to abortion and illegitimacy are related to sex, with mothers' and girls' views showing similarities, and fathers and boys recommending similar courses of action on the question of premarital conception.

Boys and girls seemed to find it easier to communicate with mothers than fathers, and maternal-child relationships appear to be easier and closer. This may partly explain why mothers have a more active role as sex educators within the family.

8

SEX EDUCATION IN SCHOOL

There is no comprehensive review of the pattern or nature
of sex education in schools, which makes it difficult to
say whether or how the topic has been dealt with in the
past. There is little doubt that, until recently (and
even now in many schools), teachers felt that their
responsibility to provide sex education was only a
responsibility if parents failed to carry out this task.
Sex education in schools was only necessary as a second
line of defence if the mothers and fathers could not or
would not provide the information themselves.

PROBLEMS OF DEFINITION

Defining sex education is more of a problem now than it
was in the first half of this century. Then the majority
of schools dealt with reproduction in science or biology
lessons, and the information was passed from teacher to
pupil in the shortest possible time. Sex education, if
it was acknowledged as such, was simply the presentation
of the basic biological facts of reproduction.

There are now probably as many definitions of sex
education as there are people who have tried to define it.
Harris (1974), for example, concludes that: 'sex
education can never be a "subject" on the timetable,
taught by experts ... it should be obvious that sex
education is a function of the entire curriculum.'

The Department of Education and Science financed in
1974 a small pilot study of teachers' attitudes to sex
education in some of the schools attended by the young
people in the pilot study (1975). Most of the head
teachers and teachers talked to in connection with this
study, although they had different views on the boundaries
of sex education, agreed that it was something more than

122

the presentation of the details of human physiology and
reproduction in biology:
> 'I can tell you why there's a rise in the number of
> abortions and illegitimate babies and promiscuity;
> they watch TV all the time and sex education is over-
> done. At 10 or 11 you should be prepared to answer
> their questions, it's the showing of pictures that's
> the problem. Sex education should not be put on the
> timetable as a subject. The biology teacher does
> animal and plant and vegetable reproduction, but as a
> church school, the religious side of it is more
> important. Our sixth commandment is "Thou shalt not
> commit adultery" and we teach that extra-marital sex
> is out of the question. We have corporal punishment
> here and I make no bones about it.'

Different viewpoints were given by two other head
teachers:
> 'There is a very great need for sex education in the
> right context - but one must teach the psychological
> and social context as well as the facts. I hope to
> build up an honest appraisal of sex education and
> teach the spiritual and psychological effects of sex.'
> 'Human relations is the key: child to child and man
> to man. You can't have a lesson on that. That's one
> of the aims of the school, to create decent relation-
> ships. But there aren't any lessons on it, it's part
> of the atmosphere of the school.'

Obviously morality and social values are considered by
these teachers to be an integral part of sex education.
This is particularly important because head teachers
control the curriculum, and therefore define sex education
to a large extent. In some schools information will take
second place to morality. In other schools information
will be paramount. But whichever way it is, information
giving cannot be 'value free'. Alongside the information,
young people are given the values and opinions of those
who teach them, even if they are not acknowledged as such
by the teachers. One of the difficulties for teenagers
is that 'learning' about sex involves adjusting to information and values - even if they are only evident in the
fact that the teacher was 'embarrassed' by teaching the
facts of life:
> 'I think the teachers were embarrassed themselves, and
> we were embarrassed because they were - it's catching!'

This chapter explores the context within which sex
education is offered at school, and the young people's
reactions to it. We show that the question is no longer
whether or not they receive sex education in school (as
it was ten years ago in the Schofield study), but whether

it is presented at an appropriate stage in their development. We also consider whether sex education is full
enough to enable young people to cope with their personal
and sexual relationships, remembering that these occur
within the context of earlier puberty and are likely to
involve earlier sexual experiences.

The only guide there is to whether sex education is
provided more often now than it was in the past is to
compare our findings with those of Schofield (1965, p.102).
In 1964, 47% of boys and 86% of girls said that they had
had some sex education in school. In this study, 87%
of the boys and 97% of the girls recalled being taught
something in this area. This difference may, in part, be
due to different definitions of sex education and the
different questions asked. Schofield's young people were
simply asked if they had ever had any sex education at
school. The teenagers in our study were asked if they
had had any sex education lessons in primary or secondary
school. They were then asked to check a list of topics,
and asked to say which had been included in the lessons.
The topics were: animal reproduction, human reproduction,
sexual intercourse, changes in a girl's body as she grows
up, changes in a boy's body as he grows up, the family
and parenthood, personal relationships between male and
female, masturbation, venereal disease, abortion, homosexuality, lesbianism. After the first question, 72% of
boys and 84% of girls said 'yes', they had had sex
education lessons. After the check list had been read
out to the ones who said 'no', a further 15% of boys and
13% of girls agreed that they had been told about one or
more of the topics on the list. There are two possible
reasons why they changed their minds. The mention of the
specific topics may have prompted their memories, and
second, our definition of sex education topics may have
been wider than theirs. The fact that 80% of those who
changed their minds said that they had been told about
animal reproduction is an indication that many of them
did not consider this as part of their definition of sex
education. This topic was included not necessarily
because we define it as sex education, but because it is
considered by many teachers to be the base for courses
on human reproduction. By some teachers it is still
considered to be the sum of sex education. A number of
young people also based criticisms of their sex education
lessons on the fact that they had only been told about
animal reproduction and nothing else. One boy said he
had had an argument with his biology teacher who
'continually went on' about the sex life of rabbits and
worms. He said: 'I told him I wasn't going to marry a

worm.' The teacher explained that he could not discuss
anything else because the headteacher would not allow it.
Memory, the definition of topics as sex education, and the
methodological differences probably account for a part of
the higher proportion of young people in our study saying
that they had had sex education at school. Some of the
increase, though, is almost certainly due to an increase
in the number of schools teaching the subjects.

The fact that more girls than boys said they had
received sex education lessons suggests that the pattern
found in the family (see Chapters 5 and 6) is repeated in
schools. Again, one likely explanation is that menstruation prompts the lessons. In the few schools we visited
this seemed to be the case. The first 'sex' related talk
said to be given in the schools was given to first- or
second-year girls by a representative from a sanitary
towel firm. At the end of their article, Leeson and Stein
(1964) made a plea for preparation for periods to be given
in primary school. The next section deals with this as a
prelude to considering the major area in secondary schools.

SEX EDUCATION IN PRIMARY SCHOOL

Only a small proportion (9%) of boys and girls in this
study remembered having any sex education lessons in
primary school. This could be an underestimate because
even the youngest in our group would be five years away
from primary education and might have difficulty remembering. But the figures do show that for most boys and girls
there was an increasing trend for the younger age groups
to say they had had some sex education in primary school
(6% of the 19-year-olds compared with 13% of the 16-year-
olds). This too could be a function of memory since the
19-year-olds are nine years away from the experience and
less likely to remember, but at the same time primary
schools are known to have become more interested in sex
education (Gill, Reid and Smith, 1974).

Of those who said they remembered having sex education
in primary school (140), most (71%) said they were 10 or
11 when they had the lessons, a fifth (20%) said they had
the lessons before they were 10, and the rest (9%) could
not remember how old they were. For the majority, sex
education in primary school consisted of one or two
lessons dealing with bodily changes at puberty and
animal and human reproduction. A third of them said they
had been told about the family and parenthood, and one in
five had been told about personal relationships between
males and females. For just over a third, films had

accompanied the lesson(s), and discussions had followed
the films for half of those who had them. The lessons
were usually said to have been taken by the class teacher,
and only 22 (or 16%) reported being taught by an outside
speaker.

Characteristics

Although it is a small group it is interesting to look
at their characteristics. More girls than boys reported
having primary school sex education lessons: 11% compared
with 7%; but there were no social class differences. The
age differences have already been discussed. The most
interesting differences were found to be regional, and
the range was large. One in four of the teenagers living
in the Croydon area, compared with one in fifty of those
living in Devon, said they had had sex education lessons
in primary school. This illustrates the clear metropoli-
tan/non-metropolitan difference which emerged here, when
children living in metropolitan districts were found to
be more likely to say they had had sex education in
primary school than those living in non-metropolitan
areas (12% compared with 6%).

It looks as if the most important factors determining
whether a child receives sex education at primary school
is the area in which they happen to live, and whether
they are female.

Reactions to primary school lessons

Although many teenagers found it difficult to remember
how they felt about their primary school lessons (15%),
a quarter of them (26%) said that they had found them
interesting and useful. One boy who said the lessons
had been about 'conception, mechanics of reproduction,
the idea of marriage and a certain amount of morality',
went on to say that he had been:
    'very impressed by the way they were done - it was
    clear and he [the teacher] spoke without embarrass-
    ment.'
Among the rest, 9% said the lessons were 'alright' or
'just another lesson - nothing special', and the remaining
young people had criticisms like 'they weren't full
enough', 'didn't have enough details', or 'were boring'.
Although a proper evaluation of sex education in primary
school would need to be carried out with children nearer
the age of eleven, these recollections give some indica-

tion that when it is part of the curriculum it is appreciated.

SEX EDUCATION IN SECONDARY SCHOOL

Reactions to sex education in secondary school will
obviously vary depending on what information a child has
previously been given. It will also depend on the age
and stage of development, and the attitudes to sex already
partially formed from earlier information. As one young
man put it:
    'They taught me all I wanted to know at the time.'
Another said:
    'I thought I could have told them a lot more, but I
    suppose they didn't know how much you understood, and
    it was alright for some in the class.'
    Although many of these teenagers had had lessons at a
variety of stages in their school careers, it was possible
to look at the age at which they remembered having their
first lesson. Table 45 shows the ages for boys and girls
of lessons in secondary school. Both boys and girls had
a mean age for their first sex education lessons of around
13 years; for boys it was 13.2 years and for girls it was
13.0 years.

TABLE 45 Age of first sex education lesson in secondary
school, by sex

Age	Boys	Girls
	%	%
11	12	19
12	19	19
13	21	20
14	19	21
15	11	13
16 plus	5	4
No sex education	13	4
Number (= 100%)	771*	770**

  * 11 excluded because inadequate answers.
 ** 4 excluded because inadequate answers.

    Although the mean age of first sex education lessons in

the 12 areas studied varied between 12.8 years and 13.4
years, there was no significant difference between the
mean ages in the metropolitan and non-metropolitan
districts. It would seem that those young people who had
sex education lessons in secondary school had their first
lesson around the age of 13.

Lesson content

One lesson on reproduction at the age of 13 would not, in
most people's view, indicate that adequate information
about sex was being provided. But this was how one in
ten (10%) of the young people in this study remembered
their sex education in school when asked how many sex
education lessons they had had. A further 20% said that
they had had two or three lessons during their school
careers, and three-fifths (59%) remembered having a series
of lessons. Nine per cent did not have sex education
lessons, and 2% could not remember how many they had had.
   There were no differences in the proportions of boys
and girls having a series of lessons, but there were
differences between types of schools. Children in state
schools were more likely to remember having a series of
lessons than children who attended public or private
schools (60% compared with 48%). Since sex education has
apparently become more widespread in recent years, it
might be expected that the younger age groups in this
study would be more likely to have had a series of
lessons and less likely to have had single lessons than
the 19-year-olds. But the data do not support this.
There is no difference either between the mixed and
single sex schools, where both groups were as likely to
remember having a series of sex education lessons.
   If a school presents a series of lessons on sex
education, it is an indication that the subject is being
taken seriously. There is, of course, a difference
between a series of lessons dealing simply with animal
reproduction and a series which deals with reproduction,
birth control, VD, and all topics related to sex. Some
indication of the differences in topics is available from
the data. For the 92% (1,424) young people in the sample
who had had some sex education in secondary school, human
reproduction was the most common subject on the curriculum,
and 78% of all the boys and girls said they had been told
about this on at least one occasion. The least common
topics were lesbianism and homosexuality, which had been
mentioned to 18% and 20% of the young people respectively.
Table 46 shows the frequency with which topics were said
to have been mentioned in school.

TABLE 46   The proportion of young people who said they
had been told about specific topics in secondary school

	Male	Female	All
	%	%	%
Animal reproduction	62	75	69
Human reproduction	73	83	78
Sexual intercourse	65	66	65
Female puberty	59	77	68
Male puberty	61	60	61
Family and parenthood	36	44	40
Personal relationships	43	43	43
Masturbation	28	19	23
Venereal disease	56	57	57
Abortion	31	33	32
Homosexuality	22	17	20
Lesbianism	18	17	18
No sex education in secondary school	13	3	8
Number (= 100%)*	773**	772***	1,545

   *   Percentages add up to more than 100% because more
than one topic was mentioned by some young people.
  ** 9 excluded because answers inadequate.
 *** 2 excluded because answers inadequate.

Boys and girls were as likely as each other to say
they had learned about sexual intercourse, male pubertal
changes, personal relationships, VD, abortion and
lesbianism. Girls were more likely to say they had
learned about animal reproduction, human reproduction,
changes in the female body at puberty, and the family and
parenthood. The boys were more likely to say that they
had learned about masturbation and homosexuality. The
differences between age groups suggest that the younger
members of the sample were more likely to say they had
learned about all the topics with the exception of animal
reproduction and female puberty. The 19-year-olds were
as likely to have learned about animal reproduction in
school as the 16-year-olds.

Some of the topics, like sexual intercourse, abortion,
homosexuality (male and female), changes in a boy's body
at puberty, family and parenthood, and personal relationships, the younger groups were much more likely to say
they had been told about in school. Confirmation of the
answers given by the 16-year-olds in this study may be
found in the National Children's Bureau study carried out

in 1974 (Fogelman, 1976). These results would seem to
suggest that secondary schools have become increasingly
conscious of the wider nature of sex education in recent
years.

TABLE 47 Proportions of young people in each age group
who said they had been told about specific topics in
secondary school

	16-year-old	17-year-olds	18-year-olds	19-year-olds
	%	%	%	%
Animal reproduction	70	68	68	70
Human reproduction	82	82	73	76
Sexual intercourse	73	70	61	59
Female puberty	69	72	66	64
Male puberty	66	64	58	56
Family and parenthood	44	46	39	32
Personal relationships	48	47	40	37
Masturbation	25	28	23	18
Venereal disease	60	60	56	51
Abortion	37	37	32	22
Homosexuality	26	21	20	13
Lesbianism	22	20	19	11
No sex education in secondary school	7	9	10	8
Number (= 100%)*	349**	403**	403**	390**

 * Percentages add to more than 100% because many young
   people mentioned more than one topic.
** 11 young people in all excluded because they gave
   inadequate answers.

One surprising finding is that the children who had
attended single sex schools appeared more likely to say
that they had been told about most of the topics listed
than those who had been to mixed schools. There used to
be a feeling that single sex schools did not pay so much
attention to sex education, whereas the mixed schools felt
it more appropriate because of exposure to the opposite
sex. This does not seem to have been true for these
teenagers. Although some of the differences are not
statistically significant, on nearly every topic a higher
proportion of those attending single sex schools said that
they had been told about it in school. The topics which
did show significant differences were animal reproduction,
human reproduction, VD, abortion, homosexuality and
lesbianism. Table 48 shows the relative proportions.

TABLE 48   Proportions of young people in mixed and single
sex secondary schools reporting on sex education topics

	Pupils attending mixed schools	Pupils attending single sex schools
	%	%
Animal reproduction	73	80
Human reproduction	73	88
Sexual intercourse	70	75
Female puberty	73	77
Male puberty	65	69
Family and parenthood	44	42
Personal relationships	46	49
Masturbation	25	27
Venereal disease	60	65
Abortion	33	39
Homosexuality	19	26
Lesbianism	18	22
No sex education in secondary schools	10	7
Number of young people (= 100%)*	943**	451**

* Percentages add to more than 100% because more than one
topic mentioned by some.
** 11 young people excluded from this table because
answers inadequate.

From these data it would seem that girls, those who
had been at school more recently, and those attending
single sex schools, are more likely to have been informed
about a wider range of sex education topics than boys,
those who had been at school a longer time ago, and those
attending mixed schools.

SUBJECT TEACHERS AND SEX EDUCATION

In the past, biology, science and physical education
teachers were the ones who traditionally took sex education
lessons.   Other subject teachers involved were domestic
science teachers because of their connection with home-
craft, and religious knowledge teachers who dealt with the
moral aspects of sex and marriage.   For the young people
in this study who said they had received some sex
education in secondary school, biology teachers still

figured prominently as sex educators. Over half (53%) of
these young people said they had been taught about sex by
them. No other subject teacher or specialist came anywhere near this. Outside speakers accounted for the next
largest group (22%), and this includes 7% who said they
had had their lessons from visiting doctors, nurses and
family planning specialists. Other outside speakers
included health visitors, sex education counsellors and
sanitary towel representatives. Only 9% of the young
people said that their religious education teacher had
dealt with sex education, but this may in part be because
they did not perceive morality as sex education.

In 9 of the 12 areas studied, about two-thirds of the
young people said their lessons had been taken by a
biology or science teacher. In the other three areas the
pattern was different. One of these areas seems to have
replaced the biology teacher with a visiting outside
speaker, whose job it was to visit most of the schools
giving talks specifically on sex education. She had
taught 69% of the young people in that area who said they
had had sex education lessons. In another area, one in
three of the young people said they had been taught by
the biology teacher (33%) and nearly a third (30%) by an
arts subject teacher. In the third area, half of the
young people said they had been taught by biology and
science teachers (55%) and nearly a third by outside
speakers (30%). These were three areas known (from
pamphlets produced by the local education committees and
personal knowledge) to have concerned themselves with
sex education and to have arranged courses for teachers
on this topic. This does not mean that other areas did
not concern themselves with sex education, but that the
teaching remains, to a large extent, in the hands of
biology and science specialists.

USE OF OUTSIDE SPEAKERS FOR SEX EDUCATION

There is disagreement amongst practitioners about the
value of using outside speakers to talk to young people
about sex and birth control. One group believes that the
teaching should be done by someone who 'knows' about the
subject - a doctor, nurse or medically qualified person.
Others argue that children should be taught by someone who
knows them and that learning should take place in a
familiar situation. There are important criteria involved
in both these arguments. It would be pointless if adolescents were given wrong or inaccurate information because
the 'familiar' teacher was not knowledgeable enough to

provide full and accurate information. On the other hand,
a properly qualified family planning specialist, giving a
one-off talk to a large group of pupils, will not be
available later if questions need to be asked or advice
sought individually.

Table 49 shows the differences in the proportions of
young people saying they had sex education lessons from
outside speakers and the levels of satisfaction expressed.
Those who had had lessons from outside speakers were more
likely to say that they were satisfied with these lessons
than those who had had lessons from their own teachers at
school. Not all young people expressed satisfaction if
they had been taught by an outside speaker, so they are
not necessarily a guarantee of satisfaction:

'Awful - she just didn't go into it properly, a diagram
here, a diagram there, and an old American film about
a boy 'phoning a girl up and asking her out. They were
much too late. They should have been shown in the
first year as soon as we got there. Now they should be
shown in primary school - as early as possible.'

However, the weight of this evidence does suggest that
the young people themselves appreciate and value visiting
speakers, and this should encourage schools to use them
more often.

TABLE 49 Satisfaction with sex education lessons by
whether taken by outside speaker

Level of satis- faction expressed by young people	Lesson taken by outside speaker	Lesson taken by teacher	All who had sex educa- tion at school
	%	%	%
Positive satisfaction	60	45	48
Neutral comment	7	15	13
Dissatisfaction	33	40	39
Number (= 100%)	261	1,018	1,279*

* 143 young people excluded because conflicting or
inadequate answers given.

SEX EDUCATION TEACHER'S SEX

The majority of young people said they had received some
of their lessons from a teacher of the same sex, but more
of the boys had lessons only from teachers of the opposite
sex, 28% compared with 19% of girls. There are a number
of possible explanations for this, but the most likely one
is that women teachers are more prepared to teach sex
education. In the same way that mothers take a more
active part in telling children of both sexes about
sexual matters (Chapter 5), so it may be that women
teachers feel it more appropriate for them to deal with
the subject in school. Amongst the teachers who were
informally interviewed during the pilot study of teachers'
attitudes, several women teachers said that in their
experience many male biology teachers refused outright to
teach human reproduction. Although there are obviously
teachers of both sexes who are reluctant to take sex
education classes, the data suggest that women taught the
subject more often than men. This does not just reflect
the relative proportions of men and women teachers, because
the ratio of male to female teachers in secondary schools
in England and Wales at January 1974 was in the region of
five to four (Department of Education and Science statistics). Like fathers, male teachers apparently take a
less active part in the sex education of schoolchildren.
In addition, the girls in the study were more likely to
have been taught about sex in single sex groups, 59%
compared with 47% of boys who were taught in single sex
groups.

AIDS TO LEARNING

Films about sex education topics can be used as a way out
of what many teachers consider a difficult lesson.
Although the films themselves may be useful in providing
information in an impersonal way, the fact that they are
sometimes shown without discussions probably makes an
impression on the adolescent mind. Not only do some
parents avoid talking about the subject, but some teachers
do too. Putting schoolchildren in a room with a projector
as a substitute for a lesson can be a clear indication of
teachers' reluctance to deal straightforwardly with the
subject. This seems to have been the case for 12% of the
young people we interviewed, who said they had been shown
sex education films without discussions of any kind. For
the rest, 42% remembered having been shown films followed
by discussions, and 46% said they had not seen any sex

education films in school at all. Young people attending
private or direct grant schools were less likely to say
they had seen sex education films in school: 38% compared
with 57% of those attending state schools. In the state
system, those attending secondary modern schools were more
likely to remember having been shown a sex education film
than those attending comprehensive or grammar schools
(62% compared with 55% and 51% respectively).

The range in the proportions in each area saying they
had seen sex education films in school varied from 30%
in Humberside to 82% in Salop. Those living in the
northern areas were less likely to say they had seen any
sex education films, 52% said they had been shown films
compared with 58% of those living in the south.

Only a few of the young people (113) could remember
the names of the films they said they had seen. These
were, 'To Janet a Son', 'Birth of a Baby', 'Susan gets a
Brother', and 'Growing Up'. But most of them remembered
the topics covered by the films. The most common subject
was the birth and development of a baby - seen by 27% of
the whole sample; the next, films about human reproduction
(22%); third was VD, remembered by 19%; and fourth, films
about puberty, seen by 18% of the sample.

The kinds of discussions the young people said they
had been involved in after seeing the films had concentrated on the film topic (this was true for 67% of those
seeing films):

'We talked about the film. [It had] already [been]
explained before we went in so there was no need for
a discussion. There wasn't much to talk about - they
just went over the film, so it wasn't much of a
discussion.'

For another 17% the discussion was wider than this and
ranged into morals and relationships:

'She asked us what we felt about the films - if we
learned anything - did we enjoy the films - did it
shock you. Did you know about that before. She talked
about drugs as well. She was very good - knew her
stuff.'

The remaining 16% were divided equally between those who
could not remember what the discussion had been about and
those who said there had not been a discussion as such,
just a talk by the teacher:

'They [discussions] were in small groups - tutor
groups - about 24 in a group. It was very flat. It
was more the teacher doing the talking with the odd
pupil chipping in.'

Books

A smaller proportion of the young people remembered having
been given sex education books to read at secondary school
(25% of the boys and 34% of the girls). The kinds of
books they remembered being given ranged from straightforward biology text books (8%) through books and
pamphlets about specific topics like puberty, VD, contraception (4%, 6% and 3% respectively) to pamphlets by
sanitary towel companies about periods and personal
hygiene (3%). Of those who did remember being given
literature on the subject(s), the majority had not found
them particularly useful; 45% said they were fairly useful
and 27% said they had not been very useful - 24% thought
they were very useful, and 4% could not remember how they
felt.
    The area differences reflected the same range as
films - from 14% saying they had been given sex education
literature in the Welsh area to 46% in the Midlands area.
Although more girls than boys said they had been given
books, amongst those who had them, there were no sex
differences in the proportions saying they found them
useful or not. However, children attending state schools
were more likely to have said they had been given books
on sex education topics (30% compared with 21% in private
schools), as were those in the younger age groups. Here
there was a trend showing that the 16-year-olds in the
sample were more likely to have been given books than the
older groups (38% compared with 22% of 19-year-olds).
Again this could be a function of memory (the younger age
groups being nearer to the event and more likely to
remember) but it could also fit in with the pattern of
the increase in interest in sex education in recent years.
    We did not spend much time on the questionnaire
investigating the young people's reactions to these 'aids
to learning'. This was partly because the pilot study
indicated that they found it difficult to recall their
reactions to the books and films in any detailed way, and
partly because the study was concentrating on other
sources of information. However, since the differences
which we did find on the basis of limited information seem
to reflect the differences in sex education as a whole,
this is probably not a serious omission.

INFORMAL OPPORTUNITIES FOR LEARNING ABOUT SEX FROM TEACHERS IN SCHOOL

Informal learning about sex from teachers can play an important part in the adolescents' learning process. For some children, being told about sex and reproduction in a large or small group can be an embarrassing and inhibiting experience. For these kinds of children, the fact that opportunities for individual discussions with teachers do not exist could be a barrier to information seeking. Also the fact that teachers offer these kinds of opportunities, outside the formal curriculum, can be a reflection of the less formal atmosphere and approach to sex education in the school. In an attempt to look at this 'informal' area of learning, we asked a series of questions about these kinds of opportunities and looked at the reasons why they were not taken up if they were offered. The questions were: 'Were you offered any opportunity to discuss sex with any of the teachers in secondary school, apart from formal lessons?'; 'What kind of opportunities were you offered to discuss sex with teachers?'; 'Did you ever take up the offer?'; 'What happened when you took up the offer?'
    Altogether 25% of the young people in this study said that they had been offered opportunities to discuss sex with teachers 'outside' formal lessons, but only a quarter of them (i.e., 6% of all young people) took up the offer. Girls were more likely to say that they had been offered such an informal discussion (28% of girls compared with 22% of boys), but they were each as likely to take up the offer. There were no area differences in opportunities offered or taken up. The most common type of opportunity they were offered was the chance to ask questions or raise problems individually outside the classroom. This was offered to 13% of the whole sample. A further 9% said that this same kind of question/problem offer was made, but only to take place during the lesson(s). Only 1% remembered help and information being offered in an open-ended way:
    'This teacher said anyone who had any problems could go and see him.'
    'The teacher that took the lessons was a counsellor and you could go to his office.'
    'Well, I mean, nuns were there all the time and we just went and talked to them if we had any problems.'
    Although the young people seemed to appreciate these offers, the fact that they were made mostly in terms of 'problems' to be discussed could be considered off-putting. Often, at that age and stage, adolescents do not have 'problems'. They may want to discuss information more

fully or they may just be 'concerned' about something.
It may not, to them, constitute a problem. This, in fact,
was the most common reason given by the 19% of young
people who did not take up the offer:

'I never had any problems so I never went.'
'Really because I hadn't any problems that I thought
needed the help of a teacher.'

Others (3%) mentioned shyness, nervousness and embarrassment as a reason:

'Well, apart from the fact there wasn't anything to
ask, I'd have been too embarrassed anyway.'

The rest, 4%, said it was not the kind of thing they
wanted to discuss with teachers:

'I never had any questions. Why ask a stranger when
you can ask your mum?'
'Because the relationship is not good enough and no
need to. [I] always discussed with parents and friends.'
'It's something you sorted out for yourselves.'

For the few (6%) who did take up the offer, a quarter
of them said they had been able to talk freely about the
matter they had raised:

'We talked about everything that we felt like,
especially in needlework - sat there sewing and
chatting about all controversial things like abortion.'
'We normally ended up boasting and laughing. One
probably doesn't learn more about sex itself, but you
do learn more about humans.'

Another 15% said they had had vague general discussions,
and as many again (16%) said the discussions had been
about specific points:

'She just explained about VD. That I didn't understand how you caught it and what it was, she explained.'

Another 18% said group discussions ensued and the rest
(25%) made a variety of comments about teacher reactions
and their own reactions:

'I felt a fool afterwards. Can't remember what I
asked her. Whenever I talk to someone I always get
mixed up.'

The question which followed this ('Were there any
teachers in secondary school you felt you could go to if
you wanted any advice or information about sexual
matters?') was aimed specifically at sexual advice seeking
and problem solving, and seemed repetitive because of the
'problem' oriented direction the opportunities question
took. But in this case, just over half of the young
people (53%) said there were teachers they felt they
could go to if they wanted advice or information. The
replies were mostly a repeat of those to the previous
question, with some additional problems described:

'There again the result was good. We had good
discussions. I remember going to Miss _____ and
telling her I was in a spot. I told her I knocked a
girl off and started hoping that she wouldn't get
pregnant. I preferred to go to her than read my books.
She told me that if she comes on with a period within
a month then okay, but if two months or more, get her
to go to a doctor. I totally object to abortion, but
if she wanted it it was okay, because we were both at
school at the time. (WAS SHE PREGNANT?) No. Miss _____
told me not to get frightened when I have intercourse
because it will shatter yourself to pieces. The next
thing she said was if I felt my sperm was going to
come, just roll off or tell the girl to get off and
stop the sperm travelling through the girl.'
'This teacher was a mature woman about 46 and she
could give me a mature answer to any problem and she
had taught a number of my family and I felt I could
trust her, in many things in school I was responsible
to her. Once I had a problem (I was very nervous, I
had a medical problem with my health). Anyway, I had
a problem, it wasn't a problem it was a childish
attitude towards girls. This woman told me to calm
down, it was a maturing stage in my relations with
girls, girls liked me but they didn't want to go out
with me as a boyfriend. That was it really.'
The reasons why those who felt teachers were available
did not go for advice or information were, again,
primarily because they felt they did not need help or
information (72%); 8% said they were too shy or nervous;
10% said they did not feel it was appropriate to ask a
teacher; and the rest just said they did not know why
they had not.
The impression left by these answers is that many
teenagers do not feel they need to use additional informal
opportunities or that teachers are not an appropriate
source of advice or information. For those who do use the
opportunities, the outcome is often satisfactory. The
fact that over half of these young people felt that they
could have approached teachers on this subject is
encouraging.

LESSONS AT SCHOOL ON BIRTH CONTROL

There are basically two types of sex education which can
be presented in school: one is part of a general knowledge
and information transmission process by which the educator
provides the pupil with an outline of facts, values and

opinions on sex; the other is an approach, much more
specific than the first, which is concerned with instruct-
ing the pupil in ways in which he can learn to deal with
his own body and emotions. The approaches are not mutually
exclusive, and often both are used in sex education
teaching. Birth control knowledge is the one practical
area where it was felt that different approaches could be
distinguished. Also, if sex educators are concerned with
the quality of life and possible consequences of sexual
experience for adolescents, then in our view it will be
necessary to provide young people with enough information
about contraception to allow them to use it wisely.

Over half the teenagers in this study (58%) said that
they had never been told about birth control in school.
For the 42% of the girls and boys who said the subject had
been discussed, the mean ages they gave for having had
lessons was 14.0 for boys and 14.4 for girls. This
difference is interesting, since Chapter 4 suggests that
on most other topics the girls had learned before the boys.
The explanation for the difference could be linked to the
fact that adolescent boys are 'expected' to become
sexually experienced at an earlier age. There were no
differences in the age at which birth control lessons
were given in state and private schools, nor between the
proportions who said they had learned about birth control
in these two types of school. There were, however,
substantial differences between the study areas. In
those areas where more teenagers said they had lessons on
birth control, the mean age figures suggest that they
also said they had been told at an earlier age. Although
it is impossible to judge the quality of the lessons from
the data, some indication is given by the number of
lessons the young people said they had, the people who
took the lessons, and the content.

Lesson content

In terms of preparing young people for the task of
controlling their fertility, it would seem to be appropriate to discuss the issues of birth control and then the
individual methods. Those who said their lessons consisted
of general discussions only would therefore seem to be less
well prepared than the others. Not everyone would agree
that this should be an aim of sex education lessons.
However, since the evidence from this survey suggests
that more young people are becoming sexually experienced
and at an earlier age (see Chapter 2), it would seem to
be increasingly important that schools should be prepared
to discuss individual methods.

TABLE 50 Area differences in proportions of young people saying they had birth control lessons at school and mean age of lessons

	% who had birth control lessons	Mean age in years when young people had lessons	Numbers in areas (= 100%)
Tyne and Wear	23%	14.5	140
Humberside	25%	14.6	125
Merseyside	32%	14.0	180
South Yorkshire	46%	14.1	123
Salop.	66%	13.9	136
West Midlands	51%	13.9	142
Gloucestershire	58%	14.0	142
Mid-Glamorgan	25%	14.7	142
Croydon	62%	14.5	121
Redbridge	43%	14.4	109
Gillingham	40%	14.4	101
Devon	35%	13.9	95
All areas	42%	14.2	1,556

Of those who said they had had birth control lessons, just over half (54%) remembered the lessons including a discussion of specific methods, and 46% said the lessons dealt only in a generalised way with birth control. The pill and the sheath were the two methods most commonly mentioned, and even these two had only been remembered as part of the lesson by 21% and 20% of the whole sample (that is, 52% and 49% of those who said they had had birth control lessons). The cap and the coil had been mentioned to 15% and 16% respectively (i.e., 37% and 38% of those having lessons), and discussion of the 'safe' period and withdrawal was remembered by 15% and 14% respectively. Only 6% of these teenagers said they had been told about all the methods of birth control shown in Table 51. This shows that relatively small numbers of young people were given specific information during the lessons in school. The numbers are too small to justify a detailed description of the kinds of advantages and disadvantages discussed.

TABLE 51 Proportions of young people learning aspects of specific birth control methods in lessons at secondary school

	Advantages discussed	Disadvantages discussed	How to use discussed
	%	%	%
The pill	16	15	11
Cap	10	11	8
I.U.D.	10	11	10
Sheath	14	14	9
Withdrawal	9	11	6
Safe period	9	11	7
Chemicals	6	7	5
Male sterilisation	10	10	7
Female sterilisation	10	10	6
Number (= 100%)	1,556	1,556	1,556

Equal proportions of girls and boys said they had their talks on birth control from visiting speakers, and girls were no more likely to say they had had a series of lessons than the boys. Altogether 41% of those who said they had had lessons on birth control had been told about it by their own biology or science teachers, a third (32%) said they had had talks from outside speakers, and another 25% said they had lessons from a range of subject teachers, including religious knowledge (10%), arts subjects (10%), and other science subject teachers (5%). Whatever their subject, women teachers (or speakers) predominated in this subject: 52% of those who were taught about birth control were told by women, 38% said that they were told by a man, 10% had lessons from both male and female teachers. As in the sex education lessons, boys were more likely to be told about birth control by a female teacher than girls were to be told by a male teacher.

REACTIONS TO SEX EDUCATION LESSONS

Although the majority of young people said they had had at least one sex education lesson in secondary school, the number of lessons, the age at which they were offered, and the content obviously varied considerably. Because of this, and because individuals have varying needs and expectations, the reactions to sex education provision were as varied as the provision itself. Table 52 shows the range of comments made by the young people in response to the question 'What did you think of the lessons in secondary school?', and separates them into positive, negative and neutral categories.

Dividing the comments into categories like this is something of a false distinction, but on the whole they did not overlap. Many of the comments contained different levels of assessment:

'They were quite useful. The contraceptives were handy. Most of the things people knew already. Our lot hadn't actually seen the birth of a baby. A lot of the boys passed out. It was a bit embarrassing I think. I think it should have been introduced earlier.'

'We tended to think that they tended to rely on the basic facts and they never really showed us a birth, and in fact we were put off because they seemed to concentrate on animal reproduction, just throwing in a few lessons on human reproduction. It wasn't until we were in the fifth year that we saw a birth and learned about pregnancy and the details.'

'Very frank and in a relaxed atmosphere. Perhaps I was lucky - there was no sniggering. Asked questions freely. We had a tape of two people who had had VD talking to each other about it. It was really good.'

'It wasn't what it was cracked up to be because most of what they said most people knew already - we had it in the fourth year and it should be in the second and third year. Let's face it, if you don't know it by the time you're 15....'

TABLE 52   Evaluation of sex education in secondary school, by sex

	Males	Females	All
	%	%	%
Positive comments (Good content, useful information	26	25	26
(Interesting topic/lesson	24	28	26
(Good atmosphere/teacher	4	5	4
(Knew most of it, but filled in some gaps	10	6	8
Neutral: Alright - just another lesson	16	17	17
(Limited content/usefulness, not enough detail	18	22	20
(Useless - boring	13	9	11
Negative comments (Just a laugh: did not take it seriously	13	8	10
(Just not very good	10	9	10
(Embarrassing	3	9	6
Some good, some bad points	4	5	4
Other comments	4	6	5
Number answering (= 100%)*	647	726	1,373**

* Percentages add to more than 100% because more than one category of answer given by some young people.

** 183 excluded because did not have sex education lessons in secondary school or gave inadequate answers.

When the comments had been allocated to one category, 45% of the young people had made mainly positive comments about their sex education lessons, 36% had made mainly negative comments, and 12% were identified as neutral, unenthusiastic comments, and 7% made comments which could not be categorised in this way. A social class analysis of the teenagers in these categories suggested that working-class teenagers were less likely to assess their sex education lessons critically (34% of them gave negative or critical evaluations compared with 40% of middle-class teenagers). This seems understandable since they are less likely to have learned from their parents, and school lessons are more likely to be their first 'authoritative' source of information.

There were no differences between the proportions of boys and girls making positive or negative comments. Interestingly, the area differences did not reflect the expected pattern. In the three areas from which a high proportion of young people reported having sex education of a 'different' kind, it was likely that there would be a higher proportion of positive comments. In fact, the reverse seemed to be the case - more positive comments were made by young people from areas where fewer young people had had any sex education. But even this was not consistent. Positive or negative comments about sex education in school would seem to be a reflection of something other than the number and content of lessons received. Although there are obviously many factors affecting reactions to sex education, our feeling at this stage is that there are two which are probably more important than others. The first is how much *accurate* information young people have been given before they have the lessons. The second, and linked to this, is the age they have the lessons. There is little doubt that physical maturation is occurring earlier. Beginning sex education lessons at 13, 14 or 15 when the mean age of menstruation is 12.5 years means that the information is not being geared to the stages of adolescent development. The chapter on sexual experience suggests that a fair proportion of young people are becoming sexually experienced before they are 16. Lessons on birth control in ' the fifth or sixth form are therefore likely to be too late to be of use to these teenagers.

SUMMARY

From the data it appears that boys are more likely to say they have had sex education in school now than they were

ten years ago. The position for girls has not changed
as much.

A small proportion of teenagers (9%) remembered having
sex education in primary school, and although not all of
them could remember what they felt about the lessons, a
third said they remembered them being very good and
useful. Add to this the criticism that secondary school
lessons came too late and the evidence that puberty begins
earlier now, and primary school sex education begins to
look like a priority.

In secondary school the majority of young people are
taught sex education by biology and science teachers,
with outside speakers playing an important part in some
of the areas. Lessons on birth control were remembered by
under half the teenagers, but very few of them remembered
being taught specifically about advantages, disadvantages
or how to use individual methods. Reactions to and satisfaction with sex education lessons are difficult to
explain. There are indications that working-class
children 'appreciate' the lessons more, possibly because
they are less likely to have been told anything by their
parents. On the other hand, middle-class children appear
to relate more easily to teachers in terms of finding
them more approachable. The comments from the young people
suggest that there is room for improvement in terms of
the age at which lessons are provided, the amount of
detail and topics discussed, and teacher presentation.

9

HOME AND SCHOOL

When parents were asked what they thought the best way was
for young people to learn about sex, over half of them
(51%) said that lessons at school were the ideal. When
they were asked specifically about sex education lessons
('Do you think boys/girls should be told about reproduction in primary school? What about secondary school?'),
only 4% said that they thought children should not be
told about reproduction in either primary or secondary
school. Not all those in favour agreed with it unhesita-
tingly. Their worries included concern that it was
'done properly' by a 'good' teacher and that some 'ideas'
should not be put into their children's heads. One
reservation was that it should not be taught too soon.
Some parents seemed apprehensive at the possibility that
sexual information might be given at what they considered
to be too early an age. This could be one explanation
for why parents are so often not the first people to tell
their children the 'facts of life', and also why schools
do not more often begin sex education lessons before the
age of 12 or 13. One of the main concerns of head
teachers introducing sex education into the curriculum is
that parents' views will raise objections. In this chapter,
parents' views of sex education in school are examined
after the young people's relationships with their teachers.
In this way we hope to throw some light on the problem of
effectiveness of sex education in schools.

TEACHERS AS A FIRST SOURCE OF INFORMATION

Since half of the parents interviewed said that lessons
at school were the best way for young people to learn
about sex, we look at teachers as a first source of
information and the young people's feelings about this.

147

In the sample as a whole, 25% of the boys and 24% of the girls said that they had first learned about 'babies' through lessons at school. Middle-class girls were less likely to have first learned in this way than the others (17% of them compared with 29% of working-class girls, 24% of middle-class boys and 26% of working-class boys). On the topic of sexual intercourse, working-class girls were the ones most likely to say that they had first learned about this in lessons at school (41% compared with 26% of working-class boys, 27% of middle-class boys and 28% of middle-class girls). So for between a fifth and a third of all social class groups, school is the first source of information on one or both reproduction topics. The data show that where school was the first source of information about reproduction and sex, the teenagers were less likely to express satisfaction with the way they had learned than those who had first heard about these things from their parents. However, they were less likely to express dissatisfaction than children who had first learned from their friends.

TABLE 53 Young people who first learned about sexual intercourse at school, from parents, and friends, by how they felt about the way they had learned

	Friends	School	Parents
	%	%	%
Very satisfied	20	30	47
Satisfied	25	27	18
Dissatisfied	55	43	35
Number (= 100%)*	629	453	175

* Base numbers are less than totals naming each source because some comments made by young people about the way they learned about sex could not be classed by degree of satisfaction.

Since satisfaction is related to source, it is worth looking in more detail at expressed satisfaction with sex education lessons and teacher-pupil relationships. The evidence presented in Chapter 8 suggests that the working-class teenagers in this study were more likely to say they were satisfied with the sex education lessons they had had, but less likely to relate to teachers in terms of approachability. Those who first learned about babies at school were more likely to make positive comments about the sex education lessons they had had than those who had

first learned elsewhere. Class differences in this group
suggest that middle-class girls were more likely to be
critical of the lessons than other groups. This may have
been because they had higher expectations than the others,
since most of the criticisms were about too little information or that it was given too late:
    'I think they could have gone into more detail a bit
    younger at secondary school, and have given us an
    outline at the primary school.'
Since we know that working-class children were less
likely to learn about sex from their parents, their
relationships with teachers as their first 'authoritative'
source of information about sex may have some influence
on the way in which they absorb this information. The
fact that they may be less likely to feel they could
approach teachers may restrict the amount or quality of
the information they acquire. Since we believe that
education cannot be value free, and that when teachers
impart information about reproduction and sex they also,
consciously or subconsciously, pass on their own attitudes
to sex, the effect this has on those who are hearing the
information for the first time may depend upon the
relationships they have with each other.
    Some evidence exists (Hargreaves, 1967) which suggests
that more working-class children are alienated from
'learning' by an educational system which 'labels' them
as less intelligent. Research has also been done which
suggests that they are less likely to 'relate' to teachers
because teachers are, for the most part, middle class and
speak and act in ways which are outside the experience of
working-class children (Bernstein, 1971). If this is so,
we might expect working-class children to accept less of
what they learn about sex at school, so that school will
not 'compensate' for the greater parental reluctance to
discuss sex with them. Sex education in school will not
necessarily fill the gap left by parents, and the only
source for acquiring information at relevant stages and
in sufficient detail will be peers.
    Once again it is difficult to claim that relationships
were 'measured' in any sense, but the teenagers' feelings
about their teachers and their perceptions of the teachers'
feelings about them were explored (they were asked, 'How
did (do) you feel about your teachers during the last two
years at school?' and 'How did (do) the teachers feel
about you during the last two years at school?'). These
feelings about teachers could be categorised into five
(almost mutually exclusive) types: those who felt teachers
regarded them favourable (37%); those who had mixed
feelings, saying some teachers liked them and some did
not (26%):

'Well, some teachers were very nice. Some you could
talk to and they'd listen, some you didn't get on well
with, some didn't really want to know.'
'It was peculiar because you either got on great with
some teachers or you never got on with them at all -
there was no in between.'
A third category felt that the teachers 'approved' of
them more during their last two years at school than they
had earlier (17%):
'They were better than they had been before - they
treated you differently because you were older.'
A fourth category remained neutral and said they had not
felt anything in particular (12%):
'They were alright. I can't remember most of them,
you just forget about them.'
A fifth category had felt the teachers' active disapproval
or disinterest (10%):
'I felt they wasn't really bothered about what you did
most of the time.'
'Terrible. (WHY?) They seemed to - well, they didn't
like me and I didn't like them.'
Some of the expected class differences did appear in
cross-analysis, with working-class boys feeling less able
to say that they had got on well with their teachers (29%
compared with 41% of middle-class boys), and more of them
saying they felt neutral or had definitely not got on
well with their teachers (26% compared with 19% of middle-
class boys). There were no differences between the
proportions of working- and middle-class girls who felt
that they had got on well with their teachers (40%
compared with 42%). Working-class boys were also less
likely to say that their teachers had regarded them
favourably (25% compared with 35% of middle-class boys)
in their last two years at school, although this could
have been affected by their school-leaving age. Many of
the comments here reflected perceived differences in
their own and the teachers' attitudes towards work, and
since many adolescent boys (and girls) see much of what
is taught as irrelevant, this is not unexpected:
'A menace, I expect. I used to take fishing books to
read in technical drawing.'
'Oh, God. I got on well with some but didn't with
others. I don't know, they never told me. I didn't
get on too well with some, because I didn't have time
for homework, being busy here. (DO YOU KNOW HOW THEY
FELT ABOUT YOU?) Some thought I could have done a lot
better than I did and I wasn't trying hard enough.'
'When I said I was leaving only one wanted me to stay
on, that was the maths. teacher because I was really

good at them. I don't think the other teachers could
have been bothered, they were glad to see me leave.'
These comments indicate that attitudes towards work are
an important part of teacher-pupil relationships.
Confirmation of this can be found in Hargreaves (1972,
p.198-218). If teacher-pupil attitudes to 'learning'
coincide, there is more likely to be a reciprocal and
meaningful relationship, through which values, attitudes
and information are transmitted. This does not mean that
those young people who have 'good' relationships with
teachers will behave differently. But it could mean that
working-class boys are less likely to listen or engage in
discussions with teachers about sex. If we add to this
the fact that working-class boys are less likely to stay
on at school (80% of working-class boys in this study had
left school by the time they were 16 compared with 43%
of middle-class boys), there is less chance of them
having discussions with teachers simply because they are
not at school so long. If young people stay on into the
sixth form when teachers often begin to treat pupils more
as equals or adults, there is a greater chance that they
will be able to discuss sex more freely with them.
     Although working-class boys are no more or less likely
to say they had sex education lessons in school than
other boys, they are less likely to feel that teachers
are approachable and less likely to feel that the teachers
liked or approved of them. They are also more likely to
leave school at 16 and to have less opportunity, therefore, of talking to teachers about sex or birth control
in an 'adult' way. The working-class boys who had first
learned about reproduction in lessons at school were
slightly less likely to say that they liked their
teachers, although the numbers were too small to show
significance (29% compared with 38% of middle-class boys,
45% of middle-class girls and 35% of working-class girls).
     If the teacher-pupil relationships of those who first
learned about sex from lessons at school are explored,
this pattern is substantiated. Over half of the working-
class boys (56%) who had first learned about sex in
school said that they did not know how the teachers felt
about them or expressed indifference, compared with a
third of the other groups (31% of middle-class boys, 36%
of middle-class girls and 33% of working-class girls).
The same difference occurred in relation to how they had
felt about their teachers. Fifty-five per cent of
working-class boys had mixed feelings, were indifferent
or made negative comments, compared with 44% of middle-
class boys, 39% of middle-class girls and 45% of working-
class girls.

These findings on class differences in teacher-pupil
relationships are supported by findings from other studies
(Hargreaves, 1967; Willmott, 1966). Willmott suggests
that schools are inevitably removed from working-class
culture: 'In a sense all schools are dedicated to the
"Protestant ethic"; all try "to turn you into something
you are not"; all are out of sympathy with the working-
class community. Teachers represent the middle-class
attitudes and enforce middle-class values and manners.'

PARENTS' VIEWS OF THE SCHOOL'S ROLE IN SEX EDUCATION

Primary school

Less than half (46%) of the parents interviewed thought
that sex education should be taught in primary schools
when they were asked outright ('Do you think boys/girls
should be told about reproduction in primary school? What
about secondary school?'). But when they were asked about
specific topics (see Table 54) a further 22% agreed that
lessons on these subjects should be included in the
primary school curriculum. Of those who thought this was
too early to begin learning about reproduction, most
expressed the opinion that childish innocence should be
preserved as long as possible:
    'It's nice to be innocent - life's not the same when
    they know the harsh facts of life.'
The subjects suggested spontaneously by the parents who
did agree with sex education in primary school were mainly
limited to reproduction (if they answered yes to the
question 'Do you think boys/girls should be told about
reproduction in primary school?' they were asked 'What do
you think they should be told at this stage?'). Nearly
half of them (48%) suggested human reproduction; just over
a third (36%) mentioned animal reproduction, and a few
(3%) thought that lessons should include some mention of
morals and relationships. When they were asked directly
about specific topics, nearly all the parents agreed that
animal reproduction should be taught at the primary school.
Table 54 shows their response to other topics and the
differences between mothers and fathers.
    As Table 54 shows, fewer fathers had reservations about
most of the topics, although not all these differences
were statistically significant. This is consistent with
the findings in Chapter 6, which show that fathers believe
that they should take a smaller part in their children's
sex education at home. As their desire to be involved in
discussions with children, particularly their daughters,

decreased with the intimacy of the subject, it is not
surprising that more of them should agree with an alternative source of learning. The greater reservation shown by
the mothers is probably inspired by their concern not to
accelerate their children's development, or because they
wish to deal with the subject themselves at that stage.

TABLE 54   Subjects parents thought should be taught in
primary school

Topic	Mothers	Fathers
	%	%
Animal reproduction	91	84
Where babies come from	51	69
Sexual intercourse	15	31
Changes in a girl's body as she grows up	48	54
Changes in a boy's body as he grows up	43	50
The family and parenthood	39	45
Personal relationships between male and female	23	27
Masturbation	10	16
Venereal disease	10	16
Abortion	6	11
Homosexuality (male and female)	8	15
Birth control	6	10
Number of parents (= 100%)*	126**	116***

* Percentages add to more than 100% because some parents
  mentioned more than one topic.
** 60 mothers excluded who believed none of these subjects
  should be taught in primary school.
*** 47 fathers excluded who believed none of these subjects
  should be taught in primary school.

In spite of the fact that many parents saw the schools
as a helpful or potential source of information, there was
a fairly low level of awareness amongst them about what
actually happened in the schools. More than a quarter
(28%) of the parents had no idea whether or not their
child had received any sex education in primary school,

and fathers were more likely to say they did not know than
mothers (36% compared with 21%). Most of the parents who
said that their child had not been taught anything about
reproduction in primary school were happy with this situation, but some of them (29%) did say that they thought
some instruction in this subject should have been given.
The reasons they gave for wishing the subject to be taught
at this stage were that they thought it necessary as a
preparation for growing up or transferring to secondary
school. The parents who said they did know that their
child had been given some instruction in the subject (12%)
mostly agreed that it was a good thing, as long as the
content of the lessons was restricted to basic reproduction. Some expressed satisfaction that the subject had
been broached in a tentative way. If the catalogue of
topics recalled by the young people themselves as having
been taught in primary school is a guide to what happens
in primary schools, then the schools hold similar beliefs
to the parents, or adjust their teaching to take account
of parental fears. On the evidence of the young people,
schools give the same priority to topics as parents at
the primary stage, and teach animal and human reproduction
(without sexual intercourse), developmental changes at
puberty and occasionally family and parenthood and personal
relationships.

On the whole, parents seem cautious about the introduction of sex education at primary school, when, as far
as they knew, it did not already occur. Over half of
those parents who knew that lessons had been given were
unenthusiastic about their child having had them. The
overall impression is that parents, whilst approving of
sex education in school, maintain a somewhat cautious
approach to its introduction at the primary level.

Secondary school

Parental enthusiasm for the subject increased when the
question of sex education in secondary school was broached,
and nearly all of them (96%) agreed with its being taught
at this level. Increased approval, however, did not seem
to be linked to greater awareness of what their own
children had been taught at this stage of their education.
Almost three-quarters (72%) of these parents said they
did not know what their children had learned in sex
education lessons at secondary school. Of those who did
know, all reported basic reproduction, about a fifth
mentioned venereal disease, a sixth said vaguely 'animals',
and less than a fifth mentioned sexual intercourse or

puberty. No other subjects were mentioned in any significant numbers.

Over half the parents did not know which subject teacher had taken the lessons; biology teachers were named by a quarter (28%), and outside or visiting speakers by 6%. Science, games and head teachers were mentioned by others. The parents thought that the lessons had been given at ages (on average, 13.1 years for boys and 13.2 years for girls) which were in line with their hopes: that is, not too early. (They were asked, 'Did (own child) have any sex education lessons at school? How old was he/she then?' They had previously been asked, 'How old should they be when they are first told about reproduction and sexual intercourse?') In spite of the lack of detailed knowledge about lesson content, the majority of parents said that they approved of the lessons their children had had. Only 10% of them reported dissatisfaction, most of them complaining that the lessons had not been full enough. One mother reported that she had written to the local newspaper to complain about the attitudes of local headmasters; when she was asked what she thought of the sex education her daughter had received, she commented:

'[It was] very bad. I wrote to the paper about it. There should be more. I had sex education lessons when I was at school during the 1940s, and I approve of them. My husband and I watched some sex education lessons, on television late at night, that they were proposing to show in schools, and we thought they were very good indeed. The three local primary school headmasters published in the paper a declaration that these films would not be shown in their schools. I wrote to the paper, saying that these headmasters were 20 years behind the times, that I wanted my children to have sex education lessons in schools, and that they had done me nothing but good. My friends all thought my letter was very good when it was published.'

Subjects parents thought should be taught in secondary school

Compared to the subjects which parents thought should be taught in primary school, the secondary school topics they listed were wider ranging. Unprompted, one in six parents mentioned sexual intercourse, venereal disease or birth control. When they were asked about specific topics, over three-quarters (79%) thought that animal reproduction should be taught, and only a minority (between 12% and 18%) thought the subjects of human reproduction, pubertal

changes, family and parenthood, and personal relationships
should *not* be taught. Abortion and birth control were
considered appropriate subjects by 70% and 76% of the
parents, but less than two-thirds of the parents approved
of including masturbation, homosexuality and lesbianism
(62%, 64% and 61% respectively).

Social class

The numbers of parents who did not feel that sex education
should be taught at the secondary level were too small for
differences to emerge. It might have been expected that
since working-class children were less likely to have been
told about reproduction at home, their parents might be
more likely to say that the subject should be taught in
school; but there were no differences on whether there
should be sex education at school, or on the topics which
parents thought should be included. Parents of both
classes were equally in favour, although their reasons for
wanting it may have been different. Mothers and fathers
were also equally likely to say they agreed with sex
education in secondary school, but when the figures were
analysed by sex and class, middle-class fathers were more
likely than either working-class mothers and working-class
fathers to say that they thought sex education should be
taught in primary school (80% compared with 64% and 62%;
68% of middle-class mothers thought primary schools should
offer sex education). It seems that paternal willingness
for the subject to be taught combines with a middle-class
tendency to want to introduce the subject at an earlier
age, to make this group more likely to be in favour of
early introduction of sex education in schools.

Parental reactions to sex education in secondary schools

When parents were asked what they thought, in general,
about young people having sex education in secondary
school, nearly two-thirds of them (64%) said they agreed
wholeheartedly with it:
    'I think it's great. This is where it should be taught.
It sinks in deeper and takes a weight from the parents.'
Only 7% said they disagreed entirely with it:
    'I don't think it's necessary. (WHY?) Same as I said,
there's time enough to learn, they'll know in time
enough.'
The remaining third (29%) of the parents expressed
approval, but with some reservations, the most common one

being that it should not be taught too soon (12%), thus
reflecting their unease with the introduction of the
subject at primary school:

'I think it's alright if it's done in the last few
years.'

'They should only have it in Grammar school at 18, but
otherwise it shouldn't be taught.'

Other reservations were linked to the quality of presentation and teaching (7%):

'I think it's a proper development but it's got to be
carefully done - needs a sympathetic teacher and good
presentation.'

and as long as it was in addition to parental instruction
(2%):

'It's a good thing as a supplement, but not as a
substitute to the education from their parents. But
if the parents feel it's their duty, I think it's
right that the children should be taught by the
teachers.'

When they were asked if they had any worries or reservations about sex education in secondary schools, similar
concerns were expressed by a similar proportion of
parents. Two-thirds of them (65%) said they had no
worries or reservations, but this time 12% mentioned the
fact that the subject should be taught by a 'suitable'
teacher:

'The person who teaches it must be suited to the job
and mustn't be very reticent and feel it's a difficult
subject or they'll make the children feel it's a
secretive subject.'

'I have no worries other than it shouldn't be thrown
at a teacher as a part-time job, a teacher should be
warned for it.'

Second, reflecting an already mentioned concern, 8% said
they felt worried that it might be taught too early, and
6% said that it should be geared to a child's development.
Finally, a few parents (2%) again expressed the fear that
the schools would take things too far.

There is little doubt that the majority of parents
were in favour of their children being taught about sexual
topics and related subjects in secondary school, and their
reservations and worries about the way and the stage the
information should be given are ones that many teachers
and pupils would share.

Although half of the parents said that school was the
best way for children to learn about sex, and nearly all
of them said they approved of sex education in secondary
school, few of them seemed to know in any detail what kind
of sex education was provided. This may be because their

children are reluctant to discuss the subject with them,
or they are reluctant to ask, but whichever it is, the
majority of the parents seemed content to allow that
teacher knows best.

SUMMARY

The implications of these data are that since working-
class children are less likely to first learn about sex
from their parents, and their relationships with teachers
are less likely to be positive, sex education in secondary
school is not necessarily a satisfactory gap-filler. Add
to this the knowledge that lessons were not often given
before the age of 13 and the mean age of first learning
about reproduction was lower than this (10.2 years;
sexual intercourse 11.6 years), and we can be fairly
certain that schools do not fill the gap left by parents.
The way is open for friends to provide the information,
often in a secretive and guilty way, since they have
already learned that it is not a subject often discussed
by parents.
     If schools are to take on the responsibility for sex
education, it needs to be done at an earlier age. In
primary school too, children's relationships with teachers
are less likely to be inhibited because, although research
suggests that class differences exist all through the
school system, enthusiasm for learning often overcomes
them.
     Whilst it seems clear that sex education in schools
leaves a lot to be desired (nearly half of the young
people (48%) had serious criticisms or apathetic comments
to make about the lessons they had had), it is also clear
that it is the source of information most readily
accessible to change. In addition, as will be shown in
Chapter 13, many of the young people believed that lessons
in school were the best way to learn about sex, and most
of the parents agreed that school was the 'proper' place
for sex education. Although there are many problems
involved in extending sex education in schools, there
seems little doubt that most parents and children would
be in favour of increasing the amount of sex education
and extending the range of subjects. However, Gagnon and
Simon (1973) point to some possible pitfalls which should
be considered:
     Of the three effective sex educational sources ... the
     schools, to judge from available data, are the least
     effective. But they do have the virtue of being the
     only one of the three that, in the immediate future,

might become the object of self-conscious programming.
This is why recent trends towards increasing sex
education in the school systems ... ought to be
encouraged. Nevertheless ... it is equally important
that such programmes be subjected to the most critical
scrutiny .... Too quickly, programmes can become the
empty rituals that serve to lessen the anxieties of
parents and educators and, at the same time, only
reinforce the children's and adolescents' already well
developed belief in the unhealthy and hypocritical
posture of adults towards sex.
Expansion alone is not necessarily enough.

10
MY FRIEND TOLD ME

LEARNING ABOUT REPRODUCTION FROM FRIENDS

Altogether, 39% of these boys and girls said that they
first learned where babies come from by talking to
friends. The two descriptions below illustrate the
initial process for many of this group (they were asked,
'Could you tell me how you first learned where babies
come from?'):
   'It was mainly at school. We used to talk between
   ourselves and we used to make it all up. We used to
   go along by what each of us individually had heard,
   then when I was older, about 12 or 13, my mother told
   me and bought me a book. Even then I didn't understand properly, but because I couldn't talk to her I
   never asked.'
   'It's a very difficult question - probably my mother
   at 12, she told me about it, said it was time I
   learned about it, but I really learned the rest from
   friends in general, and in the Scouts from the older
   lads at camp.'
More of the boys (45%) than girls (33%) said they first
learned about reproduction from their friends. This may
reflect the points observed in Chapter 5, that girls are
told at an earlier age by their mothers. Many of the
young people also said they had first learned about sexual
intercourse from their friends (51% of boys and 34% of
girls), and since fewer first learned this from their
parents, it looks as if friends move in to fill the gap.
This seems even more likely when we see that friends
featured less in relaying information about menstruation.
A previous chapter showed that the majority of girls had
first been told about periods by their mothers. In
consequence, only 15% of girls had first learned about
periods from their friends.

In addition to discussing the first time they heard about reproduction, the young people were asked which related topics they had ever discussed with their friends. Table 55 shows a high level of discussion for sexual intercourse and personal relationships for both boys and girls.

On all topics except three (the family, female puberty and personal relationships) boys are more likely to discuss them with each other. They are also more likely to discuss most of them with girls than girls are with boys. This may be a reflection of the fact that, on the whole, girls are more likely to be told about and discuss these subjects with their mother and to be slightly better catered for in the school setting. There is also an implication here that a few girls discuss these things with several boys, and the data suggest that this is so. Some of the girls in the study (24%) had discussed the less common subjects, male puberty, masturbation, abortion and homosexuality, with boys. They were more likely to be middle-class girls and to be sexually experienced; 29% of middle-class girls said they had discussed these topics with boys, compared with 20% of working-class girls, and 27% of those who said they were sexually experienced compared with 20% who said they were not. The articulate, experienced girls are the ones most likely to discuss these topics with boys. In this sense, and for these topics, the peer group is not necessarily acting as a source of information but simply as an agency for the discussion of information and ideas. But for other young people there is evidence that where family fails, friends fill the gap. There is, however, an alternative view. Gagnon and Simon (1973, p.117) maintain that the peer group acts in a way that no other source of information can: 'The continued advantage of peer groups as sources of sex education is that they can do what very few schools can even begin to do - relate sexual learning to sexual experience.' Since Simon and Gagnon believe that none of the other potential sources of information (i.e., parents, schools, media, medics or religious personnel) is capable of successfully teaching the young about sex, the peer group, because it is involved with the experience itself, is the only 'true' source of information. Although this view is not backed up with data in their book, it becomes more convincing if we look at our data on whom the teenagers said they had talked to most often about sex, and whom they had found most helpful when learning about sex. Over half the boys (59%) and a third of the girls (31%) said that they had talked most often about sex to friends of the same sex. This is by far the largest

TABLE 55 Topics discussed with friends, by sex

Topic discussed	MALES			FEMALES		
	Discussed with male friend	Discussed with female friend	Discussed with any friend	Discussed with female friend	Discussed with male friend	Discussed with any friend
	%	%	%	%	%	%
Animal reproduction	30	15	32	23	11	26
Human reproduction	56	36	60	51	29	56
Sexual intercourse	83	57	86	69	49	77
Female puberty	54	31	59	55	19	58
Male puberty	45	26	50	36	18	40
Family and parenthood	35	32	45	46	27	52
Personal relationships	57	45	64	63	44	69
Masturbation	53	21	55	32	20	38
Nothing discussed	11	31	34	12	39	42
Number (= 100%)*	782	782	782	774	774	774

* Percentages add to more than 100% because many young people had discussed more than one topic.

group - mother came next for girls (28% said they talked
to her most often), but for boys the second most common
'person' was a group of female friends. Table 56 shows
the proportions of boys and girls who said they talked
most often to particular people.

TABLE 56   People teenagers said they had talked to most
often about sex

Talked to most often about sex	Males	Females
	%	%
Friends same sex	59	31
Friends opposite sex	19	7
One friend same sex	15	25
One friend opposite sex	15	19
Mother	9	28
Father	7	4
Male teacher	4	1
Female teacher	1	5
Number (= 100%)*	782	774

(Males: 80 for first four rows; Females: 65 for first four rows)

* Percentages add to more than 100% because some young
people named more than one person.

It is clear from Table 56 that both boys and girls
talked most often to their peers about sex. This is not
particularly surprising, but if these figures and the
figures in Table 57, showing the one person teenagers
named as the most helpful when it came to learning about
sex, are looked at together, then the value of the peer
group takes on a different aspect.

A similar pattern repeats itself in Table 57 as in
Table 56. More boys named other boys as the most helpful
person they had talked to, and girls named their mothers
most often. Once again, fathers seem not to have been
mentioned very often by boys or girls. But more than
that, friends are emerging as an important and helpful
discussion source.

If we return to an exploration of sources of information and levels of expressed satisfaction, the peer group
does not appear as a satisfactory source of information,
nor is it considered to be the 'best' way to learn about
sex by very many young people (the interviewer asked:
'Looking back, what do you feel now about the way you
learned about sex?').   On the question of where babies
come from, the level of satisfaction was highest among

TABLE 57   Person teenagers found most helpful when
learning about sex

Person found most helpful		Males		Females	
		%		%	
Mother		7		22	
Father		4		2	
Same sex friends	Peers	21	47	10	46
Opposite sex friends		4		1	
Same sex friend		8		11	
Opposite sex friend		8		9	
Fiance(e)/husband/wife		2		8	
Older sibling		4		7	
Male teacher		9		2	
Female teacher		3		6	
Doctor		–		1	
Other person		3		5	
No one person		17		12	
No-one was helpful		7		3	
Not talked to anyone		3		1	
Number = 100%)		782		774	

those who had first learned from their parents: 48% of
boys and 36% of the girls who had learned in this way
said they were very happy with this method of learning:
   'Good, because I've got relations in the family I can
   talk to freely - problems came up from talks we had
   and I sorted them out with the family.'
But less than a fifth said they were very satisfied when
they had first heard where babies come from from their
friends.
   'Prefer to learn it from my friends. I don't know
   really - if your mum's going to tell you she's going
   to tell you, but I prefer to learn it from my friends.'
Table 58 shows the variations in the levels of satisfaction.
   Satisfaction was also highest amongst the group who
had first learned about sexual intercourse from their
parents. Half the young people who learned in this way
said they were very satisfied. However, of those who had
first learned about sexual intercourse from friends, only
one in five of the young people said they were very satisfied to have first heard about it in this way. Those who
had first heard about sexual intercourse from lessons at
school expressed a level of satisfaction between these

TABLE 58 First source of information about reproduction, by sex and how felt about way learned
about sex

Satisfaction with way learned about sex	MALES First learned from: Friends	School	Parents	FEMALES First learned from: Friends	School	Parents
	%	%	%	%	%	%
Very satisfied	19	29	48	17	29	36
Satisfied	29	38	29	24	25	22
Dissatisfied	52	33	23	59	46	42
Number (= 100%)*	280	170	106	242	170	239

* Base numbers are less than totals naming each source because some comments could not be classed
by degree of satisfaction.

TABLE 59 First source of information about sexual intercourse by sex and how felt about way learned about sex

Satisfaction with way learned about sex	MALES First learned from:			FEMALES First learned from:		
	Friends %	School %	Parents %	Friends %	School %	Parents %
Very satisfied	21	28	58	19	31	42
Satisfied	25	31	16	25	24	19
Dissatisfied	54	41	26	56	45	39
Number (= 100%)	380	192	50	249	261	125

* Base numbers are less than totals naming each source because some comments could not be classed by degree of satisfaction.

two, and they ranked second also on the question of
reproduction, when a third said they were very satisfied
to have learned where babies come from through lessons at
school.

The comments below illustrate the vague way some of
the young people learned about reproduction from their
friends, their feelings about it, and their suggestions
for the best way to learn about sex:

'Just gets passed around. My parents had never said
anything to me, it just gets passed around with the
friends, doesn't it? We never had any sex education
lessons at school and that. Wish I'd have been told
properly at school. I just wish anyone had told me
properly, at school or my parents. (THE BEST WAY TO
LEARN ABOUT SEX?) At school, in factual lessons.'

'Secretive, just among the mates I used to hang around
with. It used to be a bit of a laugh, just talking
about it. It's an important topic now, I suppose. It
was slow, vague, I think, until I started biology
lessons. I think you learn most of if from older
friends who know a bit more than you. (AND THE BEST
WAY TO LEARN ABOUT SEX?) I would say films, because
I would think a lot of people would be embarrassed if
you blatantly talked about it. In a darkened room
people might feel more secure. If you start teaching
at six it's better, people aren't embarrassed, they
don't really care about it then. Whereas, if you're
16, people get embarrassed. (MIXED OR SINGLE-SEX
GROUPS?) Mixed. (WHY?) Sex is between males and
females and it's pointless separating them. (SEX OF
TEACHER?) I don't think it matters. (AGE OF TEACHER?)
Young. (WHY?) I don't know about this really, but if
they're younger they might understand young people
better. I don't think they'd be so embarrassed to talk
about it. I think if you have a younger teacher, he
or she'll probably be having sex and they'll be able
to explain it better. (HOW OLD SHOULD PEOPLE BE WHEN
THEY START TO LEARN?) Eleven or twelve.'

'I don't know, I suppose it were at school. I always
thought women had footballs up there until somebody
told me. (CAN YOU REMEMBER WHO TOLD YOU?) No, it
were just some of the kids at school. (WHAT DO YOU
FEEL ABOUT THE WAY YOU LEARNED?) Same as everybody,
you find out from others. I would have liked to have
been taken to a cinema and had a right good day at it
and learn everything there is to know. (BEST WAY TO
LEARN?) Doing it, I suppose, unless they had a theatre
for a day, like I said.'

'I wouldn't know, probably at infants' school, but

that's probably on a very basic scale, to say the
least. Infants, or very early juniors. (HOW DID YOU
LEARN THERE?) Playground chatter. When I think of it
now, it was a bit of a funny way to learn - I just
picked it up. I don't know how I learned all that!
I think people should be learned about it - but not
when they're too young. (AT WHAT AGE?) I think they
should learn about periods first, because that's what
they first get - about 12 I think. And about the rest
at 13 I suppose, if you could, discussion rather than
literature - but that's really difficult to do. (WHY?)
At that age it's a joke. (AT WHAT AGE SHOULD PEOPLE
LEARN?) Well, sex is a progression. As far as your
questions have gone previously, you learn at about 10
and you're growing all the time. I would say, as far
as the real aspects of sex go, at about 14 or 15, but
it depends into what depth you go. (MIXED OR SINGLE-
SEXED GROUPS?) Separate. (WHY?) Just from my own
personal experience, I couldn't have done it in mixed
groups - but all my information stems from individuals,
not groups. I think it would be a bit farcical, cause
embarrassment. You don't get many sincere, intelligent
people at that age who are prepared to sit down and
talk about sex. (SEX OF TEACHER?) Male for male,
female for female. (AGE OF TEACHER?) As young as
possible. (WHY?) Well, from just my experience, the
younger the teacher has been, the better the contact
has been. The younger he is, the younger his views
will be, he's not going to be the old stickler.'

FRIENDS AS A SOURCE OF INFORMATION ABOUT BIRTH CONTROL

Friends were also registered as the most common point of
reference for talking about birth control. Two out of
every three teenagers said they had talked to one female
friend about it, and 61% said they had discussed birth
control with a male friend. There are differences within
the types of peer group referred to by boys and girls.
Boys consistently named other boys throughout the three
levels of talking to, talking to most often, and the
person most helpful. Table 60 shows this, and also the
fact that for girls, mothers supported or took the place
of the peer group in the 'talked to most often' and 'found
most helpful' categories. The only 'outsider' (i.e., non-
peer grouper) for boys is the male teacher, who ranks
second in the list of people most helpful to talk to about
birth control.

TABLE 60   Groups and people teenagers discussed birth control with in order mentioned most often

	MALES	%	FEMALES	%
Talked to ever about birth control	Male friends	71	One female friend	80
	One male friend	70	Female friends	69
	One female friend	56	Mother	62
	Mother	31	One male friend	51
Talked to most often about birth control	Male friends	39	Female friends	24
	One female friend	14	One female friend	20
	One male friend	12	Mother	17
	Female friends	9	One male friend	16
Found most helpful to talk to about birth control	Male friends	20	Mother	15
	Male teacher	9	Female friends	14
	One female friend	8	One female friend	13
	One male friend	7	One male friend	7

SUMMARY

This section illustrates the conflict between friends as
a source of information and friends as a testing ground
for ideas, knowledge and values. There is a relationship
between first learning about reproduction and sex from
friends and expressed dissatisfaction with the way learning
had taken place. At the same time, young people use the
peer group for discussion more frequently than any other
source, and acknowledge that they have found it useful.

11

FRIENDSHIPS AND
LEISURE ACTIVITIES

Schofield felt that his research demonstrated that
teenage groups were one of the most important influences
on teenage sexual behaviour (1965). So, in an attempt to
identify the sorts of young people who had the greatest
peer group attachment, a series of questions was asked in
this study about friendships and activities outside the
home. The largest proportion of young people (38%) said
that they saw most of one friend of the opposite sex
(including fiancé(e)s or husband/wife) in their spare
time, and one in five said that they saw most of a friend
of the same sex in their free time (the question was:
'Thinking of your friends and relatives, but leaving aside
your mother and father, who do you see most of in your
free time?'). This does not mean that they all had
exclusive friendships and saw no one else, but might be
said to reflect a preference for single relationships.
The remaining young people showed a preference for group
activities and friendships - 25% saying they spent most
of their free time with a mixed group of friends, 21%
spending it with a group of friends of the same sex, and
4% spending it with a group of friends of the opposite
sex. It is meaningless, of course, to try to divide
teenagers into types of this kind without looking at the
other important variables of age and sex. Social habits
change with age, as Willmott demonstrated in his study of
adolescent boys in Bethnal Green (1966). Table 61 shows
this change and how it compares for boys and girls. It
demonstrates that they both move from group to single
friendships as they get older, but at different stages.
    The girls are more likely to say that they see most of
one boy friend from an earlier age, and less likely to
spend their free time with a group of girls. The boys
tend to spend more of their time with a friend or friends
of their own sex.

TABLE 61   People boys and girls see most of in their spare time by age

Who see most of	16	17	18	19	All
BOYS	%	%	%	%	%
Male friends	28	27	27	24	26
One male friend	31	22	17	13	21
One female friend (includes fiancée and wife)	13	26	34	36	28
Mixed group of friends	24	28	26	29	27
Others (includes siblings and other relatives)	29	31	28	24	27
Number of boys (= 100%)*	181	213	188	199	781**
GIRLS					
Female friends	22	17	14	14	16
One female friend	26	22	20	13	20
One male friend (includes fiancé and husband)	38	47	51	57	48
Mixed group of friends	20	24	20	29	23
Others (includes siblings and other relatives)	31	22	28	26	27
Number of girls (= 100%)*	170	189	220	194	773**

*   Percentages add up to more than 100% because some gave more than one category.
** 1 boy and 1 girl excluded because answers inadequate.

The places where they met their friends most often also showed different habits for boys and girls. Over a third of the boys (37%) said they met their friends most frequently in the pub, compared with 23% of the girls. Nearly half (46%) of the girls said that their commonest meeting place was their home or their friend's home, compared with 30% of the boys. A small proportion (6%) of both boys and girls said that they loitered on street corners or around the town when they went out with their friends. In the main, the rest met most often in clubs and discotheques (12%). Age was, of course, an important factor in where time with friends was spent. The proportion of those who spent time in the pub naturally increased

with age - although it is interesting to note that one in
four of the 17-year-olds said that that was where they met
their friends most often; also 11% of the 16-year-olds.
Conversely, the number who said they spent most time with
friends in their own homes decreased with age - nearly
half of the 16-year-olds (45%) said this was the place
they met their friends most frequently, compared with less
than a third (32%) of the 19-year-olds. There were no
class differences, but those who were married or engaged
were more likely to meet their friends in their own homes.
Work status also influenced where people met. The ones
who were unemployed were less likely to meet in the pub
and slightly more likely to meet in their own homes than
those who were at work or college. This would seem to be
a natural outcome of not having money. The people who
were still at school were less likely to meet their friends
in the pub (16% compared with 33%) but equally likely to
meet in their own homes.

The amount of time spent with friends is likely to be
influential in the kind of discussion young people have,
as well as the places they go to. It is also difficult
to record accurately. The young people in this study were
simply asked how many times they went out in a typical
week. The mean number of times for boys was higher than
for girls (4.3 compared with 3.4).

The pattern of peer group relationships which emerges
in this study is different for boys and girls but changes
for both as they get older. Girls tend to spend less
time with their female peers and to begin single heterosexual relationships at an earlier age. The boys appear
to have a more male-oriented and outgoing pattern of
relationships which persists until a later stage.

Social class

There were few differences between middle-class and
working-class boys, in terms of time spent with the
different peer group types. Middle-class boys were more
likely to say they saw most of a mixed group of friends
than working-class boys (33% compared with 23%). Girls
of both groups were more likely to say they spent their
time with one male friend than boys were to say they did
with one female friend. Apart from the indication that
middle-class boys spend more time with a mixed group of
friends, these differences only reflect the different
patterns for boys and girls. An analysis of the people
they said they felt closest to shows that there were no
differences between middle-class and working-class boys,

but the girls were more likely to say they felt close to
one friend of the opposite sex. The differences between
middle-class girls and working-class girls (more middle-
class girls saying they felt closest to one friend of the
opposite sex, 34% compared with 26% of working-class girls,
and less likely to say they felt closest to siblings,
fiancés and husbands) can be explained by the fact that
working-class girls were more likely to be married or
engaged (22% compared with 15% of middle-class girls).
Being sexually experienced does not seem to change this
pattern.

SEXUAL EXPERIENCE AND FRIENDSHIP

Schofield (1965) found that sexually experienced boys were
more likely to be members of a group of boys and sexually
experienced girls were more likely to be part of a mixed
group. In this study the findings were more in line with
an expected courtship pattern. Boys who were sexually
experienced were more likely to most often spend their
free time with a female friend than boys who were not
sexually experienced (40% compared with 12%). Also
sexually experienced girls were most likely to say they
spent most of their free time with one friend of the
opposite sex (including fiancé or husband). Two-thirds
of the sexually experienced girls said this compared with
32% of the girls who were not sexually experienced. This
was true for all ages.
    Sexual experience also had an effect on whom the
teenagers felt closest to, as might be expected. Sexually
experienced boys of all ages were more likely to say they
felt closest to one friend of the opposite sex than boys
who were not sexually experienced; the latter were more
likely to say they felt closest to siblings. Sexually
experienced girls were more likely to say they felt
closest to one male friend than girls without experience;
but girls who were not sexually experienced were more
likely than non-experienced boys to say they felt closest
to one friend of the opposite sex. So, although sexual
experience changes close relationships, within the sexes,
the differential patterns (between the sexes) remain.
Table 62 shows these relationships and the differences
between boys and girls.
    It is interesting that age made no difference to this
pattern amongst the boys when sexual experience is held
constant. Sexually experienced 16-year-old boys were as
likely to say they felt closest to one friend of the
opposite sex when the wife/fiancée category is included

TABLE 62 People to whom boys and girls felt closest (excepting their parents) by sex and sexual experience

Felt closest to	MALES		FEMALES	
	Sexually experienced	Not sexually experienced	Sexually experienced	Not sexually experienced
	%	%	%	%
One friend of same sex	13	18	13	24
One friend of opposite sex	31	13	37	24
Spouse or fiancé(e)	6	-	30	4
Friends of same sex	8	13	3	7
Friends of opposite sex	2	1	1	1
Friends of both sexes	5	7	1	4
Siblings	18	26	8	23
Others	17	22	7	13
Number (= 100%)	420*	309*	352**	364**

* 13 experienced and 13 non-experienced boys excluded because answer inadequate.
** 5 experienced and 13 non-experienced girls excluded because answer inadequate.

(31% of sexually experienced 16-year-old boys said this
compared with 26% of 19-year-olds; or 39% of 19-year-olds
if the wife/fiancée category is included). Age did make
a difference to the girls - 57% of sexually experienced
16-year-old girls said they felt closest to one male
friend, their husband or fiancé, compared with 70% of
19-year-old girls. The really important difference lies
between those who were experienced and those who were not,
and not between age groups. Those who were experienced
had progressed to heterosexual, non-family relationships,
whereas those who were not had close relationships with
friends of the same sex and siblings. This would seem to
be more to do with maturation and progression than
chronological age or friendship patterns. The fact that
those who were not sexually experienced showed a greater
attachment to their family (parents) is demonstrated by
an analysis of a question about whom teenagers felt had
been the most important influence in their lives. Those
who were not sexually experienced were more likely to say
that their parents had been the most important influence
for them, irrespective of age or class. Table 63 shows
the proportions of young people saying this, by sex,
class and sexual experience.

The middle-class groups were slightly more likely to
name their parents than working-class teenagers, but the
main differences occur between the sexually experienced
and those who were not.

These findings are consistent with the suggestion that
sexual experience is more a function of maturity and
close relationships than it is of group membership, and
that group membership or attachment is a function of age
and sex. Adolescents do move away from family dependence
and influence as they get older, to form relationships
with members of the opposite sex - and sexual experience
is simply part of this new relationship. It is
impossible to say that group membership of a particular
kind encourages teenagers to become sexually experienced,
since this study did not explore pre-experience friendships. Affiliations, group membership and leisure habits
do change as young people gain experience, but this would
seem to be part of the normal 'courtship' pattern, rather
than the result of any particular 'group' attachment.

One further finding is of interest because it demonstrates the extent to which teenagers felt they were
conforming to a peer group norm. They were asked what
proportion of unmarried boys and girls of their own age
they thought had had sexual intercourse. Tables 64 and
65 show that those who were sexually experienced were much
more likely to say that all or most young people did, than
those who were not sexually experienced.

TABLE 63 Proportions of teenagers who said parents or friends were the most important influence on their lives, by sex and social class

Most important influence	MIDDLE CLASS				WORKING CLASS			
	MALE		FEMALE		MALE		FEMALE	
	Sexually experienced	Not sexually experienced	Sexually experienced	Not sexually experienced	Sexually experienced	Not sexually experienced	Sexually experienced	Not sexually experienced
	%	%	%	%	%	%	%	%
Parents	53	65	51	66	48	60	43	63
Friends	13	10	21	9	21	9	23	13
Spouse or fiancé(e)	3	-	7	1	3	-	10	1
Others	18	11	13	16	17	15	13	9
No one person	13	14	8	8	11	16	11	14
Number (=100%)*	151	147	137	134	254	157	192	212

* 10 young people excluded from this table because answers inadequate.

TABLE 64 Young people's perceptions of proportion of unmarried boys of own age who have sex before marriage, by sex and sexual experience

What proportion of unmarried boys have sex before marriage	MALE		FEMALE	
	Sexually experienced	Not sexually experienced	Sexually experienced	Not sexually experienced
	%	%	%	%
All or most	76	27	80	52
About half	17	25	14	24
Some but less than half	7	44	6	21
None	-	4	-	3
Number (= 100%)	431*	308*	339**	333**

* 10 and 16 boys excluded because answer inadequate.
** 1 and 14 girls excluded because answer inadequate.

TABLE 65 Young people's perceptions of proportion of unmarried girls of own age who have sex before marriage, by sex and sexual experience

What proportion of unmarried girls have sex before marriage	MALE		FEMALE	
	Sexually experienced	Not sexually experienced	Sexually experienced	Not sexually experienced
	%	%	%	%
All or most	69	22	73	35
About half	22	24	19	27
Some but less than half	9	48	8	36
None	–	6	–	2
Number (= 100%)	423*	306*	356**	363**

* 2 and 14 boys excluded because answer inadequate.
** 18 and 44 girls excluded because answer inadequate.

The evidence here for 'conformity' amongst the sexually
experienced is overwhelming. In which direction the
conformity occurs is less clear, because attitudes and
beliefs about others are often brought into line with
individual behaviour. It is possible, therefore, that the
sexually experienced teenagers said they thought others
had sex before marriage to justify their own actions to
themselves (and possibly to the interviewer). However,
very few of the teenagers who were not sexually experienced
said that no unmarried teenagers had sex before marriage,
and therefore the conclusion that by becoming sexually
experienced, teenagers are conforming to the norm, is not
out of place. Class differences reflect different class
beliefs and behaviour. Working-class boys were more
likely to say that all or most unmarried boys had sex
before marriage, 65% compared with 42% of middle-class
boys. There were no differences between the proportion of
middle-class and working-class girls saying all or most
unmarried girls had sex before marriage (56% compared with
51% of middle-class girls). Analysis by age also showed
that beliefs reflected what happened amongst age peers.
With both boys and girls, more of the older teenagers
said that all or most unmarried young people had sex
before marriage. In each male age group the proportion
of boys saying that all or most unmarried boys had sex
before marriage corresponded with the proportion of the
sexually experienced. But more of the younger girls than
were experienced thought that all or most unmarried girls
had sex before marriage. This evidence does suggest that
young people saw sex before marriage as a common event,
and in this sense, if they were sexually experienced, or
became so, they were only doing what they believed most
unmarried teenagers did.

Learning from friends and sexual experience

The two preceding chapters showed that those who had
first learned about sex from their friends were less
likely to express satisfaction with the way they had
learned than those who had first learned from their
parents. Schofield suggested that there was a strong
association between friends as a first source of information and teenage sexual experience (Schofield, 1965, p.165).
His findings are corroborated to a certain extent in this
study, but some changes have taken place. Table 67
compares his findings with ours, and shows that whilst
girls who first learned about sexual intercourse from
friends are more likely to be sexually experienced, this

TABLE 66 Proportion of boys and girls who were sexually experienced and who thought all or most unmarried boys/girls had sex before marriage, by age and sex

	MALE				FEMALE			
Age:	16	17	18	19	16	17	18	19
% sexually experienced	31	50	65	74	22	39	52	67
% who said all or most unmarried boys/girls had sex before marriage	34	50	63	72	36	51	61	62
Numbers in each age group*	181	214	188	199	170	190	220	194

* Base numbers for percentages are slightly less than totals in age groups because some answers were inadequate.

TABLE 67 First source of information about sexual intercourse, by sexual experience, compared with 1964 findings

First source	1964*			1974		
	Parents	Friends	School	Parents	Friends	School
MALES	%	%	%	%	%	%
Sexually experienced	24	31	32	55	60	42
'Inceptive'**) Not sexually	24	40	24	45	40	58
'No experience') experienced	52	29	44			
Number of males (= 100%)***	42	281	50	49	382	196
FEMALES	%	%	%	%	%	%
Sexually experienced	9	21	12	44	62	39
'Inceptive'**) Not sexually	42	47	28	56	38	61
'No experience') experienced	49	32	60			
Number of females (= 100%)***	135	193	85	122	251	267

* 1964 figures derived from Schofield (1965) Table 10.2, p.165.

** Schofield had an intermediate category 'inceptive' for young people who had experienced some sexual activity short of sexual intercourse.

*** Young people who refused to say if they were sexually experienced are excluded from both sets of figures.

is no longer true for boys. Also fewer young people are
learning in the first instance from friends, and their
role as a source of information has been taken by the
schools. Now boys and girls who first learn about sexual
intercourse through lessons at school are less likely to
be sexually experienced than those who learn from friends -
yet the levels of sexual experience are higher. It is
interesting that Schofield's connection between sexual
experience and friends as first source, shows only if his
experienced and inceptive categories are put together.
These two categories then look like the experienced group
in our study. It is as if the greater sexual activity of
today has superimposed on the source.

SUMMARY

If the data on first learning about sex from friends are
considered again, we know that working-class boys were
more likely to say they first learned where babies come
from from friends, and were more likely to be sexually
experienced. Boys as a group were more likely to say
they had learned from friends than girls. These 'facts'
reflect part of a different pattern of learning about
sex, which is most obviously different for boys and girls,
but also illustrates a class difference for boys. The
changing social climate and relatively freer expression
of sexuality within relationships, means that all teenagers are more likely to have sexual experience before
they marry. The context within which their learning
takes place will be important for all of them, but
cannot be shown to have a causal relationship to early
sexual experience.
   Since it seems clear that friends are the first to
provide information about sex because parents do not
provide it, or because they do not provide it soon enough,
and given that those who first learn from friends are less
likely to express satisfaction with the way they learned,
the remedy would seem to lie in encouraging parents to
tell their children or to tell them earlier. But since
it has also been shown that many parents find it difficult
to carry out this task, an alternative approach would be
to try to ensure that if friends do provide information
they provide accurate information. This can only be done
by presenting basic information at an early age. Puberty
occurs earlier now, and if the trend to earlier sexual
experience suggested in this study is accurate, most
children need to be given information before they leave
primary school, and this information needs to be expanded

and developed in the first two years of secondary school.
The concept of birth control and the availability of
services for birth control advice should be introduced
no later than thirteen, even though more detailed
information might be postponed until the third or fourth
years. If this happened in schools, there would be less
chance of friends providing inaccurate or worrying
information. They would then remain as an important
source for the discussion and exchange of ideas and
experiences, but the content of these discussions would
be better informed.

12

DOCTORS, TEENAGERS
AND CONTRACEPTION

This chapter describes the way young people regarded
general practitioners and birth control clinics as
contraceptive advice and information providers. The
first part looks at the attitudes and use of general
practitioners for this purpose, and the second part at
the attitudes and use of birth control clinics for
contraceptive advice.

Whatever views are held about the appropriateness of
medical control of contraceptive advice for young unmarried people, in principle they should feel free to
visit their own doctors for birth control advice and
supplies. In practice there are problems. Embarrassment,
uncertainty about the doctor's reaction, fear that he
will break a confidence - all these can be seen as
barriers to doctors providing an unhampered service to
young people. In order to assess how truly available
general practitioners seemed to be to teenagers, we
asked a series of questions about their relationships
with their own doctors.

Young people's relationships with their doctors

The questions fell into four categories: how well they
knew their own general practitioner; how easy they felt
he was to talk to; whether they felt he had time to
discuss things with them; and whether they felt he would
tell their parents about personal matters which they had
discussed with him. All these were things which could
inhibit or encourage young people to seek advice. The
first question - how well they knew their doctor - revealed
that over half (51%) of them felt they did not know him
well, and this was more often true for boys than girls
(54% compared with 49%). The proportion saying they found

their doctor difficult to talk to was lower than this, but true for one in four of all the teenagers we talked to. On this question it was the girls who were more likely than boys to report difficulties in communication (30% compared with 19%). This is important since we know that girls are more likely to approach their doctors for advice. The reasons given by those who did find it difficult to talk to general practitioners fell mainly into three categories - those who believed that the doctor did not know them well or that they did not know him well enough to feel at ease (17%); another group (18%) who said that their doctor was unapproachable because he was either too old, too strict or too busy; and a much smaller group (2%) who gave communication problems as a reason for not finding their doctor easy to talk to:

'He's got a stutter and he just can't speak.'
'He's an English doctor but I can just understand him.' (This from a Pakistani boy)

Some of the comments made by those who felt their doctor was unapproachable are more serious, since general practitioners are now as important an agency for the provision of birth control advice as the birth control clinics (Bone, 1973, Table 2.1, p.14). They said things like:

'Well, he hasn't got time to talk, he's always too busy.'
'He's not the nicest of people to talk to. I think he would look down on me if I went to ask him for advice.'
'As I said, he's no time for you, and he's a snob.'

We should not forget, however, that criticisms of this kind came from a third of the young people, and that two-thirds (66%) said that they found their doctors comparatively easy to talk to.

Patients' perceptions of doctor approachability (in the NHS at least) must, to some extent, be governed by the belief that he is a busy man. Other studies have shown that doctors themselves feel that time is a serious problem and that they find inadequate time a frustrating element in their jobs (Mechanic, 1968; Cartwright, 1967 and 1970).

This knowledge, plus the fact that birth control was not included in the National Health Service until recently, probably influenced the young people who felt that their doctor did not have time to discuss things with them (47% of girls in the study and 45% of boys). An attempt to relate area variations in the proportions saying their doctors did not have time to discuss things with them,

TABLE 68 Regional variations in the proportions of young people saying their doctors did not have time to discuss things with them, with shortfall/surplus of general practitioners

Sample areas	% of young people saying doctor did not have time	Family Practitioner Committee areas	Percentage shortfall(-) or surplus(+) of principals*
Merseyside	60% (180)	St Helens & Knowsley	-16%
Tyne and Wear	52% (140)	North Tyneside	- 8%
West Midlands	47% (142)	Birmingham	- 1%
Salop	46% (136)	Salop	+ 3%
South Yorkshire	46% (123)	Sheffield	-11%
Humberside	41% (125)	Humberside	+ 3%
All northern areas	49% (846)	All above northern areas	- 4%
Devon	50% (95)	Devon	+13%
Kent	48% (101)	Kent	- 3%
Croydon	43% (121)	Croydon	- 2%
Mid-Glamorgan	40% (142)	Mid-Glamorgan	- 2%
Redbridge	37% (109)	Redbridge & Waltham Forest	+ 2%
Gloucestershire	34% (142)	Gloucestershire	+12%
All southern areas	41% (710)	All above southern areas	+ 3%
All areas	46% (1556)	All above areas	-

* Shortfall/surplus calculated by finding difference between actual number of doctors in area and the ratio of number of patients in area to England and Wales average list size (2,386) and expressing this difference as a percentage of the latter. Numbers of doctors and patients in each Family Practitioner Committee area were taken from unpublished Department of Health and Social Security tabulations of General Medical Services in England and Wales, 1st October 1973.

with the shortfall or surplus of general practitioners
in 1973 (calculated from DHSS figures, see footnote to
Table 68), revealed no consistent findings.

As can be seen from Table 68, in some areas like St
Helens and Knowsley, and North Tyneside where there was
a shortage of general practitioners in 1973, young people
were more likely to say that their doctors did not have
time to discuss things with them. Overall, young people
living in the north felt this to be true more often than
those living in the south (49% compared with 41%). Also,
there was a significant difference between those living
in Metropolitan and non-Metropolitan districts (49%
compared with 42%). Although the areas used in Table 68
do not compare exactly with the areas used in our study
(e.g., Devon), it seems clear that doctors working in
some areas where there is a shortgall of medical practitioners do manage to convey to young people the impression
that they are too busy to sit and discuss their problems.

There is, however, a clear relationship between whether
the young people felt the doctor had time to discuss
things with them, their level of confidence in him with
regard to personal communications, and how easy they found
him to talk to. Tables 69 and 70 show quite clearly that
those young people who felt their doctors had time to
discuss things with them were more likely to say they
found him easy to talk to, and more likely to feel certain
that he would not tell their parents about personal
matters. Table 71 shows that those who found their doctor
very easy to talk to were also more likely to express
trust in him. In an analysis of these factors the same
relationship between time, confidence and ease of communication is expressed.

TABLE 69 Relationship between time and communication

Talking to doctor	Doctor has time to discuss things	Doctor does not have time to discuss things
	%	%
Very easy	38	15
Fairly easy	48	37
Not very easy	9	42
Other comment	5	6
Number (= 100%)	659	705

TABLE 70   Relationship between time and confidence

If told doctor something personal, would he tell parents?	Doctor has time to discuss things	Doctor does not have time to discuss things
	%	%
Certain would not tell	61	47
Fairly certain would not tell	26	26
Uncertain if would tell	12	25
Other comment	1	2
Number (= 100%)	659	705

TABLE 71   Relationship between communication and confidence

| If told doctor something personal, would he tell parents? | Talking to doctor | | |
	Very easy	Fairly easy	Not very easy
	%	%	%
Certain would not tell	68	53	41
Fairly certain would not tell	22	30	27
Uncertain if would tell	10	17	32
Number (= 100%)	371	627	362

Surprisingly, perhaps, there were no social class differences in the attitudes expressed towards general practitioners. Similar proportions of boys and girls felt that their general practitioner did not have time to discuss things with them (45% and 47%), and amongst the girls those who found the doctor difficult to talk to were more likely to express uncertainty about whether he would pass on confidential matters to their parents than boys were (32% compared with 14%). Age also seemed to affect the teenagers' attitudes on this question. The younger they were, the less likely they were to say that they were certain the doctor would keep their confidences (the trend was from 42% at 16 to 60% at 19). This is likely to be a

fairly accurate assessment of what might happen, since
doctors might feel that they should give information to
the parents of 16-year-olds when they would not consider
it for 19-year-olds.

It seems likely that those young people who had been
able to establish an 'easy' relationship with their
doctor, because he had been approachable or prepared to
spend time with them, and felt they knew him well, were
more likely to feel certain that he would not reveal
personal confidences to their parents. It is also likely
that doctors who are prepared to talk to young people are
sympathetic to their problems and make it clear that they
understand the need not to do this.

Reasons for not using general practitioners for birth
control advice

To explore further their feelings about visiting doctors
for birth control advice, the young people were asked to
say what sort of things might stop them going to see him
and in what circumstances they would go to ask him for
contraceptive advice or supplies (they were asked: 'Could
you say what sort of things might stop you going to a
doctor, even though you might like his advice on birth
control?' 'In what kind of circumstances would you go to
a doctor for birth control advice?'). Over a third (35%)
said that nothing would stop them going to see their
doctors for this purpose if they wanted to, but nearly
as many (29%) mentioned embarrassment, and an eighth (12%)
mentioned confidentiality worries:

  'Well, there's always a chance that he might tell your
  parents.'
Others (7%) said that their general practitioner's attitude
would put them off:
  'His attitude - he's so cold and old-fashioned.'
  'Well, I don't like my doctor - he's very abrupt and
  I couldn't talk to him very well.'
Other points made here were that doctors were too busy for
that kind of thing (5%), and that the opposite sex of the
doctor (3%) was off-putting.

Considering the circumstances in which they would go
to a doctor for birth control advice, nearly a third (31%)
said they would go whenever they wanted information, advice
or supplies. But another 10% said they would only go if
they were married or had children, and 7% mentioned
pregnancy outside marriage as a circumstance in which they
would go to him for advice:
  'If I thought I'd got a girl in the club.'

Another group mentioned getting married as an appropriate
time to go and see the doctor for advice, but 9% said they
would never go under any circumstances.

It seems that apart from a group of young people (about
a third) who were convinced that they would freely use
their general practitioners as birth control consultants,
the reservations and situations which the others mentioned
mostly related to their own embarrassment about birth
control and the attitudes of some of the doctors. If
young people are to be encouraged to use doctors for this
purpose, work needs to be done to change these attitudes
and to help young people to overcome their reservations.

However, it should be emphasised that these findings
are based on attitude questions and not necessarily on
experience. The fact that the older age groups tended to
be less critical, and the knowledge we have that the 18-
and 19-year-olds were more likely to be sexually experienced and therefore to have visited their general practitioner for birth control advice, suggest that their
experiences are better than expectations and possibly lead
to changes in attitudes. To see if this is true, the
experiences of those young people who had visited their
doctor for contraceptive advice are considered.

Young people using general practitioners as a source of
contraceptive advice

Not unexpectedly, the majority of teenagers who said they
had visited a general practitioner for birth control
advice were girls. Altogether, 47% of the sexually
experienced girls had sought his advice (only 2% of
sexually experienced boys). Almost all of these girls
had been to their own general practitioner (93%). When
they talked about their feelings before they had been to
the doctor for advice, most of them (71%) said that they
had been very nervous or embarrassed before they went.
They made comments like:
    'It took me two months to pluck up courage.'
    '[I was] apprehensive - I wasn't sure if that was the
    thing to see a doctor about - that sounds silly now,
    I know.'
A smaller group (16%) said they had no worries about
going, sometimes because they had had a baby and felt
more justified:
    'I wasn't embarrassed - I'd lost all my shame. Well,
    it was the same doctor what done the ante-natal.'
Some (5%) said that they felt it was the right thing to
do or they had been reassured by friends:

'Quite happy, because I knew I wasn't the only one
who'd been.'
Satisfaction with the way they were treated was
expressed by three-quarters (76%) of those who had been
to their general practitioner for advice:
'Our doctor's very understanding and I trust him. I
didn't mind once we'd started talking.'
More casually:
'We had a little chat. He ripped off a prescription,
said "Try that and see how you like it. Come back in
three months."'
But some girls were not so lucky: 13% of the ones who had
been to the doctor had been given warnings and disapproval
as well as the pill:
'He just said, "I suppose I have to give it you, if
not you'll only come here pregnant. You should wait
till you've got a ring on your finger."'
'There was no fuss made but he did give me a lecture
on the dangers of being promiscuous on the pill.'
The rest of the comments (11%) were mainly expressions of
neutrality:
'It was alright - just like normal.'
'Very politely.'
Two-thirds of them (67%) said that the first time they
consulted him for this purpose it was better than they
had expected. Another 25% said it was about the same as
they expected, and only 6% said the visit was worse than
they had expected.
On the whole, those girls who had been to seek medical
advice from their general practitioner had not been put
off in any way by their experiences. This may have been
because their original expectations were low, or because
they saw us as a medical organisation and were reluctant
to criticise. But whatever the reason, their reactions
to the visits seem to have been mainly favourable. The
number of boys visiting general practitioners is too
small for any meaningful analysis to be undertaken.
In spite of the overall satisfaction expressed by the
teenagers with the general practitioner service, there is
room for improvement. The characteristics of the girls
who had visited only their doctor for advice show that
they were, in the main, the older girls (76% were 18 or
over) and more likely to be married or engaged (58% of
marrieds had been, 28% of engageds and only 13% of the
single girls). It seems clear that older girls who are
married, engaged or having a stable relationship, once
they have overcome their initial nervousness, have few
reservations about using doctors for birth control advice.
The problem, if it can be seen as such, is how to attract

single girls and boys into doctors' surgeries, if that is
where birth control services for the young should be
concentrated.

Attitudes to birth control clinics

The majority of young people had heard of family planning
clinics (94%) and knew what they were for. The 98 (6%)
who had not heard of clinics were predominantly male (10%
of boys compared with 3% of girls), concentrated in the
younger age groups (13% of 16-year-olds compared with
2% of the 19-year-olds), and two-thirds of them (69%) were
from working-class families (3% of middle-class young
people had not heard of birth control clinics compared
with 8% of the working-class group). Those who had heard
of birth control clinics were asked what they felt the
advantages and disadvantages to be. Nearly half (48%)
said that the advantages of clinics for providing birth
control advice were that they specialised and knew more
about birth control. A typical comment from those who
gave specialisation as one of the advantages of clinics
for birth control advice was:
   'The fact that that is all they're dealing with,
   whereas with GP's it's just one of many - you'd be
   more likely to get expert advice.'
Another such comment was:
   'That's all they deal with, that's their speciality.
   If they don't know, who does?'
Other advantages mentioned (by 22%) related to the
preferred anonymity of clinics, that they were seen as
being more approachable and posing fewer risks to confidentiality than general practitioners:
   'Well, it's a lot easier going to them than the
   doctor. They don't know you and you don't know them,
   and it's easy to talk freely, and if you go to your
   own doctor you'll feel he might possibly tell your
   parents.'
   'For people that don't want to go to their doctors,
   don't want their doctors to know. They know they can
   get reliable advice and there's no danger of getting
   lessons in morals or anything like they do from their
   own doctor.'
One other important advantage of clinics mentioned by
11% of the young people was that they had better facilities
for tests and supplied information and pamphlets:
   'That's their job really - they do all the tests that
   need to be done if you're on the pill, but the doctor
   would just dish out six-monthly supplies and not bother

to take your blood pressure or anything.'
'They specialise. They've got the best advice,
pamphlets. They know everything. They've got time to
discuss things with you.'
From these findings it would appear that most of the
teenagers had a clear idea of the advantages of seeking
birth control advice from clinics. This is interesting
in the light of the findings later in this chapter, which
show that relatively few of them had used clinics for
this purpose when they became sexually experienced.

When they were asked to mention any disadvantages they
thought there were to the provision of birth control
advice by clinics, over a third (35%) said they did not
think there were any. A comparatively small 13% said that
they felt they were too impersonal and saw not being known
by the doctors there as a disadvantage:

'I suppose it's a bit - everyone feels a bit embarrassed,
no not embarrassed - I suppose it's a bit downgraded
to go to one of those places. It's a bit like a cattle
market. No matter who you are, you are all come for
the same thing and you're all treated the same.'

'Can't think of any [disadvantages] apart from the
fact that they like to see their own doctor about it
because maybe they'd like to talk to someone who knows
them.'

Among other disadvantages mentioned by a few of the teenagers (9%) was that everyone would know what they were
there for:

'People more or less know what you're going there for,
for that specific reason.'

A handful of young people also mentioned other reasons
like there were not enough clinics, or that they were not
accessible or sufficiently well publicised (4%), or that
the time spent waiting in clinics was a disadvantage (3%),
but on the whole more teenagers seemed aware of the advantages than disadvantages.

When they were asked to say whether they would prefer
to go to a clinic or a doctor for professional advice
about birth control, 44% chose their own doctor and 48%
chose a birth control clinic. The remaining 8% said they
would go to another doctor (4%) or made other comments
(3%) or said they did not know (1%).

The girls were more likely to choose a birth control
clinic (52% compared with 44% of the boys), as were the
19-year-olds in the sample (55% compared with 44% of the
16-year-olds) and the young people who lived in the
Metropolitan areas (53% compared with 42%). This may well
be due to the greater availability of clinics in towns.
Sexually experienced boys were more likely to say they

would prefer to go to a birth control clinic (49% compared
with 36% of non-experienced boys) but there were no differences between the girls who said they were experienced
and those who said they were not.

Four-fifths (80%) of the young people who said they
would prefer to go to their own doctor for birth control
advice said that it was because they knew him better and
could talk to him better than a strange doctor:

'I just feel I could talk to him better than any other
doctor or a strange one at the Family Planning Clinic.'
'Because they know you and I think it's more personal
and private than a clinic.'

The reason most commonly given for preferring a birth
control clinic (by 60% of those who chose the clinic) was
that they were specialists and knew more about birth
control:

'They specialise in it. I think it would be easier to
talk to them because that's what they're doing all day.'

Another reason given for preferring the clinic (by 29% of
those who said they did) was that they were more anonymous and 'confidential' than general practitioners:

'I wouldn't know them and they wouldn't know me.'

Use of birth control clinics by teenagers

The experiences of those girls who had been to a birth
control clinic for advice (21% of the sexually experienced
girls) were similar to those who had chosen to use general
practitioner services. Here, 70% found their first
experience better than they had expected, 24% said it was
about the same, and only 4% said it was worse than
expected. Again, the majority (78%) said that they had
been embarrassed or nervous before they went to the
clinic:

'I think I was a bit embarrassed in a way. When you
have to wait in there with a load of women – and
especially when all the others being called up are
"Mrs" – and then a "Miss" goes up.'

But again almost all of them (88%) said that the way they
were treated on the first occasion had reassured them:

'Very nice. They put you at ease and try to gain your
confidence – which they do.'

Some had reservations of an unexpected kind:

'Very well – as if I'd been married for six years.
They were very understanding. But I think it's too
early to go here, and you know – I've got a stable
relationship but other people could go there and
pretend they had and still get their pills.'

Only two girls (i.e. 2%) said they were treated with
disapproval:
> 'It was a bit upsetting because they could be more
> friendly than what they are. There was like an atmos-
> phere in the place and that's what made the people so
> tensed up.'

The rest (10%) said that their reception was alright
and much as they had expected. Although we did not ask
for this information, it emerged that the reason that
some girls felt better about the clinic was that their
boyfriend (or fiancé) had gone to the appointment with
them. None of the girls who had been to their general
practitioner mentioned this. It may be that if boys were
encouraged to accept their responsibility as partners in
contraceptive use, and made it clear to their girlfriends
that they were prepared to share in advice getting, more
girls would use birth control clinics:
> 'I didn't really want to go, but felt better because
> Mark was with me.'
> 'My boyfriend came with me and we both wanted some kind
> of reliable method. I suppose I was a little bit
> jumpy - but alright.'

Reasons for not using clinics

The young people who were sexually experienced but had
not been to a clinic were asked why they had not been.
The largest group said it was because they had no need to
go or did not want to go (34%):
> 'Because I never needed to - the machine in the pub is
> less embarrassing and more convenient.'
> 'Mainly because at the birth control clinic you've
> got a lot of mucking about with you - with examina-
> tions; at the doctor's I never had an examination
> since I've been on the pill (3 years).'

Another 15% said they had never thought about going to a
clinic, and 24% said they (or their partners) got advice
and supplies elsewhere:
> 'I never thought about it, the first place I went to
> was the doctor.'

A small group (5%) said they were too shy or embarrassed
to go to the clinic, and another 7% said that they did
not know where the clinic was:
> 'I don't know where it is to tell you the truth,
> they're not advertised.'

The remaining 15% could not say why they had not been, or
made a variety of other comments.
  They were also asked in what circumstances they would

consider visiting a clinic, and 22% said that they would
go if they had any worries about contraception or any
difficulties:
    'If I wanted to change the type of contraceptive or
    if my doctor advised me to go.'
Another 19% said they would go after they got married or
when they were engaged or 'going steady':
    'Perhaps when I'm married.'
    'If I was engaged and wasn't planning to get married
    for a few years, then I'd go I think.'
For some (12%) there were no circumstances in which they
would go to a clinic, and others (6%) said they would
only go if they had specific pregnancy or VD problems.
The rest said either that they would use a clinic if for
some reason they could not get supplies from their doctor
(10%), or made other comments.
    Although the numbers using clinics were small, the
characteristics of those who did use them give something
of a guide to the reasons why more young people do not go
there for contraceptive advice. Most of them were girls
(81%). Although clinics themselves often encourage male
partners to attend, nothing else in the system does. Sex
education in the family and at school is directed more
at girls, and since the most reliable methods of contraception are female methods, girls take the responsibility.
The girls were more likely to be married or engaged (25%
of all the married girls had been to a clinic, 19% of
those who said they were engaged, and only 7% of those
who were single). This is almost certainly because
clinics are seen still as places where married women go
to control their fertility. It is also partly because
going to the clinic for advice makes public their sexual
experience, going to the doctor is more anonymous in the
sense that no one (except the doctor) knows that he is
being visited for birth control advice.

SUMMARY

The characteristics of those using clinics are very
similar to those of the ones who visit their general
practitioner. Similar proportions of them said that
their experiences at the clinics had been better, the
same or worse than they expected; that is, most saying
they were better and very few saying they were worse than
expected.
    Amongst the wider group of young people (that is, all
those interviewed, not just the sexually experienced),
knowledge about the advantages and disadvantages of birth

control clinics and general practitioners for birth
control advice seemed well advised for the most part.   The
young people were almost equally divided on their prefer-
ences for attending one or the other, with girls showing
a preference for birth control clinics and boys for
general practitioners. The difference seems to be between
those who preferred anonymity and specialist doctors and
those who wanted advice from someone who knew them well
(the general practitioner). However, it is interesting
to note that when they come to the point of making a
choice, more girls visited a general practitioner than
went to a clinic (47% of sexually experienced girls had
ever been to a general practitioner compared with 21% who
had been to a clinic). It seems likely that the availability of general practitioners and the fact that surgeries
are less 'obvious' places for birth control advice has
some influence when the choice eventually comes to be
made.

13

LEARNING, SATISFACTION AND EXPERIENCE

This chapter pulls together the findings on the way young people learned about sex, their feelings about that process, and the way in which their learning had affected their behaviour in terms of sexual experience and use of birth control. It seems likely, from what has been shown earlier in the book, that there is no direct causal link between learning and behaviour. This should reassure those who feel that knowledge is dangerous and can lead young people to practise what they know before they are mature enough to know what they are doing. The fact that teenagers who said they had first learned about reproduction from friends were more likely to be sexually experienced, does not mean that if they had been told first by their parents they would not have had sex at such an early age. The fact that they were told by friends and expressed dissatisfaction with the way they learned is a much more important finding. What is crucial is that young people should feel that they have sufficient information to enable them to be involved in heterosexual relationships comfortably and confidently, whenever the occasion arises. Wagner maintains that information about sex is as important to human sexual growth and development as any other information relating to any other kind of human behaviour (in published literature from a lecture prepared for the Family Planning Association by N. Wagner given in 1973 entitled 'Should you make contraceptives available to your teenaged child?'). But there are still groups and individuals who exert pressure against early or full sex education because they feel that the information itself can lead to 'wrong' behaviour. The young people themselves showed a remarkable sensitivity and awareness of their own need for information and some of the risks accompanying its provision. When they were asked what they thought was the best way to learn about sex, over

half of them (56%) mentioned lessons at school, and many
of the comments referred specifically to the need for
information about sexual matters to be treated 'normally'
as part of life or education:

'Basics at school - in a proper, separate, regular
lesson - so that it is just part of your education.
It shouldn't be made out as something special, you
know, to say "You will not have history today you will
be having a film" - and everyone knows what it will be -
it just becomes a novelty and people laugh at it and
treat it as a joke. If it is made just a part of
general education, just growing up, the basic tools of
life, that sort of thing - I don't see why it should
be any different to teaching history - it's much more
important anyway, so why shouldn't you have a period
a week from the beginning of secondary school? People
would say a period a week was too much, but if you can
drag something like Maths, English or any typical
subject out for five years, I don't see why you can't
do it with sex. It would also make sex less stigma-
tised - people would treat it as a normal part of life.'

VIEWS ABOUT THEIR SEX EDUCATION

Lessons in school were mentioned as the best way of
learning about sex more often than any other method, and
parents were also more likely to mention this source of
information as the best way to learn. Parents themselves
were the second most frequently mentioned 'best' source
of information (37%). Altogether 72% of the teenagers
mentioned one or both of these sources. There is an
interesting division here, though, between the young
people who felt that it was more appropriate for learning
about sex to take place within a close family relationship
and those who felt it was better to learn in a less
personal setting. The two quotations below reflect these
different viewpoints:

'From your mum. I don't think it's a good idea to
have sex education in school because children get
embarrassed sitting learning things like this. I
think it's better to be by yourself. In a whole class
the teacher has to explain and the kids laugh and don't
take any interest, and some of them get embarrassed by
it and some of them get upset.'
'Straight to the point, don't mess about. Not all at
once - gradually. The best way would be in school.
You could ask your parents but you'd be too shy. I
suppose some people would say you should learn from

your parents, but I've never sat down like you see in
the adverts and had a talk about it with them.'
Some young people mentioned a combination of parents and
school, pointing to the advantages of both sources:
    'I think it should be a mixture of at home and school.
    You can't see a film at home, but you should know
    before you go to school and get more details there,
    perhaps.'
    'I think the parents ought to say, but I think a lot
    could be done in schools. I think formal lessons
    should be devoted to it and films, because a lot of
    parents don't tell their children, I would imagine.'
    'Well, I think you want to learn from parents to begin
    with. I don't think they should give you a leaflet,
    they should talk to you about it and be open about it.
    I don't think my parents were open enough. School
    should help - I've never seen one of the films they
    show but it sounds a good idea.'
Analysis of these views of the best way to learn about
sex showed that girls were more likely to mention parents
as the ideal source of information (49% compared with 26%
of boys), possibly reflecting the greater likelihood of
their having learned this way. Boys were more likely to
say that friends were the best way to learn (11% compared
with 6% of girls), although the numbers suggesting this
way of learning as the best way were small. Table 72
shows that these sex differences were maintained in an
analysis of the young people's views of the best way to
learn about sex, by sexual experience. Other differences
show that sexually experienced boys were more likely than
boys who were not sexually experienced to say that the
best way to learn was from experience, and that non-
experienced boys were more likely to suggest that films
and books were the best way to learn. Sexually experienced
girls were slightly less likely to say that parents were
the best source of information than girls who were not
experienced.
    Some differences emerged between middle-class and
· working-class boys. Working-class boys were less likely
to suggest that parents were the best way to learn about
sex (22% said this compared with 32% of middle-class boys),
and more likely to say that learning from one's own experience was the best way (16% compared with 7% of middle-class
boys). There were no differences between suggestions made
by middle-class and working-class girls as to the best way
to learn about sex.
    Moving on from the ideal source of information to the
young people's reactions to the way they themselves had
learned, it is clear that many of them felt that the

TABLE 72   Male and female views of the best way to learn about sex, by sexual experience

Best way to learn	MALES		FEMALES	
	Sexually experienced	Not sexually experienced	Sexually experienced	Not sexually experienced
	%	%	%	%
Lessons at school	55	60	54	55
Parents	24	28	47	52
Films/books	19	26	23	28
Own experience	19	4	5	2
Friends	12	10	6	6
Someone who 'knows'	8	8	8	6
None of these	7	7	6	7
Number (= 100%)*	433	322	357	376

* Percentages add up to more than 100% because some young people gave more than one source.

process could have been better. Only 23% of the teenagers expressed positive satisfaction with the way they had learned about sex (they were asked, 'Looking back, what do you feel now about the way you learned about sex?'). Another 26% said that it had been 'alright' or made neutral or unenthusiastic comments, and the rest (51%) made a variety of critical comments, some of which (15%) openly expressed dissatisfaction.

One girl had initially learned about reproduction and sexual intercourse from other girls, 'picking it up from a number of friends' when she was 11. In the same year, but later, she had had lessons in secondary school about puberty and periods from a Tampax representative, and when she was 15 or 16 had been told about reproduction, venereal disease and contraceptives by her biology teacher. When she was asked how she felt about the way she had learned about sex, she said:

'It's wrong. It's something you should know, it's part of life, something you need to know, so I think it should be given earlier, the teaching in school, like any other subject. If the majority of parents are like mine, in that they didn't say much, then I think it should be taught in school like any other subject.'

A boy, who had also learned at first from friends and who said:

'[I] picked it up in bits and pieces from here and there'

had felt that he had not had any sex education in school because:

'About the only thing I had that approached a sex lesson was from a biology master who was a bit of a hoot; laughing, he told us "Put it this way, if you put two Rolls Royces in a garage, you won't come down in the morning and find a load of Minis".'

When he was asked how he felt about the way he had learned about sex, this boy said:

'Well, I think I managed alright but maybe a little help on the way would have helped.'

One of the most frequently expressed criticisms was that not enough detail had been given when learning took place. This was mentioned by 15% of the young people:

'I think I could have been taught more. With my parents it was always "sex isn't to be mentioned" attitude.'

Other criticisms were that information had been given at too late a stage (17%), and that more openness about the subject would have been appreciated (9%):

'The way I learned I don't think it was too bad, but I

wish I could have been taught it earlier when I was
10, and that the way I had been told wasn't undercover
and hush-hush like it is amongst friends. It should
be open and not concealed.'

Preference for an alternative source was expressed by 18%
of the teenagers - 7% of whom said they would have
preferred to have learned from their parents, and 9% who
said they would have been more satisfied if they had had
lessons at school.

To summarise the young people's reactions to the way
they themselves had learned about sex, only one in four
was completely satisfied. Girls were more likely to make
critical comments than boys (53% did compared with 47%
of the boys). The boys were not more likely to say that
they were satisfied, but more likely to express indifference or neutrality (30% compared with 23% of the girls).
Comments like 'It was okay', 'It was alright', and a
general lack of enthusiasm, were more commonly heard from
boys than girls. Criticisms did not seem to be related
to sexual experience. Sexually experienced girls were
no more likely to express dissatisfaction with the way
they had learned than girls who were not sexually experienced, but they were more likely to be critical than either
sexually experienced boys and boys who were not sexually
experienced (56% of sexually experienced girls said they
were in some way dissatisfied compared with 50% of girls
not sexually experienced, 47% of sexually experienced
boys, and 48% of non-sexually experienced boys). The
fact that girls were more likely to have learned from
their parents, and that those who learned in this way
were more likely to say they were satisfied with the way
they had learned, suggests that girls as a whole have
higher expectations of their parents, and possibly of
other sources, than boys. This in turn could lead them
to be more critical of any source which fails to offer
information or offers only a minimal amount. It could
also be that girls get information from less competent
or articulate parents. There were no class differences
in the overall levels of satisfaction expressed, and this
seems to reinforce findings throughout the book, that it
is the differences between the sexes which are most
consistent and important. On the other hand, if a class
analysis of satisfaction by first source of information
about reproduction is examined, working-class boys were
less dissatisfied than middle-class boys, if they had
first learned about babies at school (32% compared with
51%). This difference between working-class boys and
middle-class boys disappeared when first learning about
sexual intercourse was considered. In this analysis there

were no differences between the two groups of boys, but
middle-class girls were more likely than middle-class boys
to make critical comments if they had first learned from
their parents. It does seem likely that satisfaction with
learning is linked to source of first learning about sex,
and that girls' expectations are higher because they are,
on the whole, told more at an earlier stage. Working-
class boys are more likely to be satisfied if they have
their first information from school, whilst being as aware
as others that friends are not a satisfactory first source.

VIEWS ABOUT THEIR KNOWLEDGE OF BIRTH CONTROL

Nearly two-thirds of the young people in the sample felt
that they had learned about birth control at the right
time (65%), but nearly one in four (23%) said that they
felt that they had learned about it at too late a stage.
One in ten of them (10%) felt that they had not learned
about birth control at the time they were asked the
question ('Do you think you learned about birth control
at the right time, too soon, too late, or that you haven't
learned about birth control?'). Although less than half
of them had had birth control lessons in school, there was
a link for those who did have lessons, between the age
they had the lessons and whether they felt they had learned
at the right time; 78% of those who had the lessons before
the age of 14 felt that they had learned at the right time
compared with 67% of those who had had the lessons at the
age of 14 or after.
    When they were asked how they felt now about the way
they had learned about birth control, nearly half the
young people (44%) expressed dissatisfaction, and the most
common complaint they registered was that they had learned
too little too late:
    'I reckon I should have been told when I was younger.
    I found out about it when I was 15. I just heard
    people talking about it, like.'
    'It was very haphazard. It was never really defined
    or taught to me. I just picked it up. It was left
    up to me.'
These kinds of comments were made by one in four of the
young people (24%). Others said they were dissatisfied
with the way they had learned because they felt they
should have learned in school (10%):
    'I never learned anything at school about them, only
    from seeing things in the pubs and barbers, and stuff
    about the pill in the papers.'

Another 9% were dissatisfied because they had 'just picked up' the information and had never really been told:

'It wasn't very good - I wasn't given any definite information, it was more of a case of picking it up here and there.'

'It was quite poor, I suppose. It was probably only by accident I did learn any detail and I wouldn't have got that if I hadn't read any books and things.'

The rest were dissatisfied because they felt they had learned from unreliable sources (3%), or they would have liked to have been told by their parents (2%).

Only one in five (19%) of the young people were completely satisfied with the way they had learned about birth control, and a further 9% said they were fairly satisfied but had some reservations:

'I'm quite happy about it, but I think there's still a bit more to learn, but I suppose I'll learn that as I get older.'

Altogether, then, 28% said they were satisfied or fairly satisfied with the way they had learned about birth control, 44% were dissatisfied, 22% were unenthusiastic, saying 'it was alright' or they 'didn't have strong feelings about it', and 6% said they could not answer because they felt they had not really learned about birth control.

Levels of satisfaction did seem to be related to whether birth control had been taught in school; 41% of those who said they had had birth control lessons expressed satisfaction with the way they learned compared with only 18% of those who did not have lessons. School and lessons were also mentioned most frequently when the young people were asked what they thought was the best way to learn about birth control (by 48%):

'At school. Someone from the Family Planning Association should go around schools and talk to people. They'd listen to them.'

'At school, at the same time as the other sex education - telling you what methods and tell you which is the best.'

(The percentages which follow do not add up to 100% because several gave more than one answer.) Doctors and parents were mentioned next, but only by 19% and 18% respectively. Reading and films featured more often as the best ways to learn about birth control than they did in learning about reproduction or sex; 17% mentioned reading and 13% mentioned films or television:

'Films and reading. If you can read something by yourself, it's informative - and if you see a film you can take it in as well. I think you have to explain explicitly about how each form of birth control works.'

Reading and films in conjunction with discussion also seemed to be favoured:

'To be given an outline first of all, then to read,
and then afterwards to discuss it if you don't
understand anything.'
Over half the young people (52%) said they had read
something about birth control. The most common forms of
literature mentioned were magazine and newspaper articles
(17%) and contraceptive pamphlets (16%). A small number
(6%) remembered reading Family Planning Association
pamphlets, and 2% mentioned school text books; 14% said
they had read something but could not remember what, and
3% said they had read advertisements and instructions in
contraceptive packets. The most common sources of
obtaining this 'reading' material were schools and
teachers (13%), and in the case of magazines and instructions, they had been bought from shops (13%). Nine per
cent had been given the literature by clinics and doctors,
and another 8% had got it from friends. The rest had
been given the literature from a variety of sources
including libraries (2%), parents and siblings (7%). The
information on birth control films was less specific, but
15% remembered seeing a television documentary, and
another 6% said they had seen something on the television
about birth control but could not remember what kind of
programme. Altogether a third (39%) of the young people
remembered seeing at least one film about birth control.
Of these, 24% said it had been very useful, 58% said it
had been fairly useful, and 18% said it had not been very
useful. Slightly higher proportions of those who had
learned (partly or wholly) through reading birth control
literature had found it very useful (33%), and fairly
useful (52%). A fairly small group had found the literature they read not very useful (15%).
   Opinions about the value of literature and films on
birth control suggest that although they are important as
the best source for some young people, for most of them
they represent a useful aid and addition to other primary
sources.
   Finally, discussion with 'someone who knows' (15%) and
friends (6%) were mentioned as the best way to learn by
a fifth of the sample:
   'Talking with friends, getting different people's
   ideas, and with grown-ups. That's mainly it.'
   'It always helps to have a session with someone who
   knows about it - a doctor or someone like that.'
Table 73 shows that once again the major differences in
opinion were between boys and girls - with boys more
likely to say that school was the best place to learn
about birth control, whilst girls were more likely to say
that parents (almost always mother) and doctors were a

TABLE 73   The best way to learn about birth control by sex and sexual experience

The best way to learn about birth control	MALES		FEMALES	
	Sexually experienced	Not sexually experienced	Sexually experienced	Not sexually experienced
	%	%	%	%
Lessons at school	53	55	42	45
Books	17	15	15	19
Films	15	14	7	14
Parent(s)	13	15	21	23
Doctor	15	9	33	20
Discussion with someone who knows	16	13	16	16
Discussion with friends	8	7	6	5
From experience	5	1	1	1
Other way	6	10	8	7
Number (= 100%)*	433	322	357	377

* Percentages add to more than 100% because many young people gave more than one answer.

more appropriate source. Sexually experienced boys were
more likely than other boys to mention doctors as the best
way to learn, but only one in seven of them did so, whilst
one in three sexually experienced girls thought doctors
were the best way to learn.

Analyses by social class did not reveal any differences
between groups of boys, but sexually experienced working-
class girls were less likely to say that lessons at school
were the best way to learn than middle-class girls (38%
compared with 50% of middle-class girls), and also less
likely to suggest films and books as an ideal source than
middle-class not sexually experienced girls (13% compared
with 23%).

Learning about birth control seems to be regarded
differently from learning about reproduction. Its more
technical aspects seem to lead young peopld to feel that
teachers, literature and films are more appropriate
sources of learning. Once the young people are sexually
experienced, doctors become a fairly important source,
for girls especially.

SOURCES AND BEHAVIOUR

Sexual experience

So far exploration of different first sources of learning
about sex has indicated that girls are more likely to
first learn from their parents and boys from friends.
Girls who had learned from friends were more likely to
be sexually experienced than girls who had learned from
their parents. Also middle-class children were more
likely to first learn from their parents than working-
class children. This might lead to an assumption that
source of learning and early sexual experience go hand in
hand. In fact, when source is held constant no class
differences appear. Table 74 shows that all class groups
who had learned about sexual intercourse from friends
were as likely to be sexually experienced. The only
significant difference to emerge here is that working-
class boys who had first learned about sex at school were
more likely to be sexually experienced than middle-class
boys who had also learned about sex at school.

Apart from this, within each social class group the
pattern is exactly the same. Those who had first learned
about sex from friends were more likely to be sexually
experienced than those who had first learned at school,
but not more likely than those who had first learned from
their parents. This lack of difference between friends

TABLE 74 Source of first learning about sex, by sex, social class and sexual experience

	Middle-class males			Working-class males		
	First source			First source		
	Friends	Parents	School	Friends	Parents	School
	%	%	%	%	%	%
Sexually experienced	54	61	32	64	47	49
Not sexually experienced	46	39	68	36	53	51
Number (= 100%)	143	31	81	214	17	104

	Middle-class females			Working-class females		
	Friends	Parents	School	Friends	Parents	School
	%	%	%	%	%	%
Sexually experienced	58	43	41	61	47	39
Not sexually experienced	42	57	59	39	53	61
Number (= 100%)	101	69	76	135	45	169

and parents as a first source is probably due to the
small numbers of each group who had first learned from
their parents. The differences between those who had
first learned from friends and those who had learned at
school present something of a puzzle. It is tempting to
suggest that if the first source of information about sex
is a friend or friends, then early teenage sexual experience will follow. But since other variables like age and
sex have been shown to be crucial in all other analyses,
it would be misleading to say this. Also to suggest
that information provision on one occasion, several years
earlier, can influence sexual activity, would be to
ignore everything that is known about cultural patterns
of behaviour. The most that should be said about first
source of information and subsequent sexual behaviour is
that they are linked insofar as they represent the
different ways in which boys and girls are prepared for
sexual activity. Neither sex is currently given as much
information as they would wish for, at an age they think
appropriate, or from a source which they regard as
authoritative. This may, on occasion, lead them to
experiment or to try to find out for themselves. But it
is much more likely that the link between learning and
behaviour reflects cultural and sexual traditions of
which early sexual experience is a part.

Birth control

Knowledge of birth control was shown to be related to
sexual experience and use of particular methods in
Chapter 3. To some extent this is inevitable, but there
is a great deal of room for improvement. The fact that
those who had had birth control lessons at school before
they were 14 were more likely to say they had learned
about birth control at the right time, suggests that
early instruction (before intercourse happens) is regarded
as more appropriate by the young people themselves. Table
75 shows that those who had the highest scores on birth
control knowledge were more likely to say that doctors
and friends had been the most useful person when it came
to learning about birth control. The findings suggest
that knowledge increases after sexual intercourse has
occurred.

TABLE 75 Mean scores on knowledge of birth control
questionnaire by person most helpful in learning about
birth control, by sexual experience

Person most helpful for learning about birth control	Sexually experienced Mean score	Not sexually experienced Mean score
Parents	4.5 (80)	3.4 (108)
Friends	4.4 (292)	3.8 (249)
Teacher	4.2 (44)	3.8 (82)
Doctor	4.8 (87)	4.4 (14)
Other sources	4.2 (111)	2.9 (45)
No single source the most helpful	4.4 (125)	3.8 (98)
No-one talked to about birth control	3.3 (30)	2.2 (88)

( ) Base numbers for means in brackets.

In spite of knowledge being linked to experience, Table
76 shows that birth control education at school does make
a difference to the knowledge young people have before
they become sexually experienced. Of those who were not
sexually experienced, both boys and girls who had had
lessons at school had a higher score on the birth control
knowledge questions than those who had not had lessons.
Sexually experienced boys who had not had lessons scored
as highly as boys who had, but sexually experienced girls
who had not had lessons had a significantly smaller score
than the experienced girls who had had lessons at school.
This evidence suggests that birth control education at
school does make a difference to the amount of birth
control knowledge young people have before they become
sexually experienced. If young people are to be prepared
for sexual relationships in a responsible way, and birth
control lessons can be shown to make a difference to birth
control knowledge, then there is no question that they
should be part of every secondary school curriculum. On
the other hand, having birth control lessons at school
did not seem to affect use of birth control amongst these
teenagers. Girls who had lessons at school were no more
likely to have always used birth control than those who
had not had lessons (38% compared with 41%), and boys who
had not had lessons at school were slightly more likely

TABLE 76 Mean scores on birth control knowledge and lessons at school by sex and sexual experience

	MALES		FEMALES	
	Sexually experienced	Not sexually experienced	Sexually experienced	Not sexually experienced
	Mean score	Mean score	Mean score	Mean score
Had birth control lessons at school	4.2 (170)	4.1 (144)	4.8 (138)	3.8 (168)
Did not have birth control lessons at school	4.3 (260)	3.3 (177)	4.3 (216)	3.0 (208)

( ) Numbers involved in each mean are in brackets.

to say they had always used birth control than boys who had
had lessons. Age is probably the intervening factor here,
since younger boys were more likely to have had birth
control lessons but less likely to be sexually experienced.
The fact that birth control lessons in school are more
likely to be part of the curriculum now than in the past
probably means that, for the older boys, lessons were not
a consideration when they first became sexually experienced.
Schofield (1965) did not ask about birth control lessons
specifically, but only two-thirds of his teenagers said
they had had any sex education at school, compared with
92% of the teenagers in this study, half of whom had had
birth control lessons.

Even though birth control use is not apparently affected
by birth control lessons, the fact that the young people
themselves felt that lessons were the best way to learn,
and that their knowledge was greater if they had had
lessons, indicates that this is one way in which they can
be helped to control their fertility, if they want to.

DOES LEARNING MATTER?

One of the basic assumptions of this study was that
learning about sex matters to each individual because
knowledge and information help people to feel that they
are able to exercise some control over their future
decisions and actions. It matters on a wider level to
society, because the degree to which responsibility for
the transmission of knowledge is taken up by institutions
reflects the care society has for its members. Although
the assumption that the way young people acquire sexual
knowledge matters seems obvious, it rarely gets an airing,
yet it is the one on which sex educationists base their
efforts to change or improve the learning process. There
is little doubt that attitudes to sex in Western societies
have changed, and that discussions of sex are more open
now than they were a hundred years ago. Whether these
changes in attitudes affect sexual behaviour or simply
reflect the changes in behaviour which are taking place,
is a question discussed by Osofsky in an article published
in 1971. He suggests that attitudes to sex may change as
a result of changes in sexual behaviour, or alternatively
that behavioural changes in sexual habits take place
because attitudes have changed. He goes on to say that
'alterations in patterns of sexual behaviour which occurred
during the early part of this century, together with the
recognition of these alterations as a result of scientific
investigations, may have preceded and contributed to present

day thinking. Attitudes may merely have caught up with existent behaviour.' He then introduces evidence from two recent American studies which suggest, he thinks, that attitudes have not only caught up with reported sexual behaviour but 'may have passed beyond them' (pp.398-9). Combining results from this study and Schofield's, there has been an increase of 250% in the proportion of girls reporting experience of sexual intercourse since 1964, compared with a corresponding increase of 170% for boys (Schofield, 1965, pp.39-40). Whilst this evidence supports Osofsky's general findings that male adolescent rates of sexual activity are not increasing as fast as female adolescent rates of premarital sexual activity, the only evidence we have about behaviour overtaking attitudes would not confirm his suggestions. The fact that more girls in this study said that they approved of sex before marriage than were actually experienced, is an indication that their attitudes were more liberal than their actions (30% of the non-experienced girls said they approved of sex before marriage).

Also, the findings reported in Chapter 11, that a higher proportion of girls said that all or most of their peers had sex before marriage, than reported they themselves had, suggest their attitudes or beliefs about others outstrip, in time at least, their own sexual involvement. Osofsky concludes his article by saying that changes in adolescent sexual behaviour could occur in either direction; that is, that rates of both behavioural and attitudinal change may begin to decline. On the other hand, he says: 'Recent data, while obviously not conclusive, suggest the possibility of quantitative increments in adolescent female sexual behaviour, and qualitative changes for both sexes.' These 'intuitions' are untestable from our data, but the reference to qualitative changes for both sexes is important. If there are to be 'qualitative' changes in adolescent sexual behaviour for both males and females, the information on which they make their individual decisions about when and how they become sexually involved will itself need to be of an appropriate and relevant quality. The evidence presented in earlier chapters suggests that for many young people, whether they had learned from parents, school or, particularly, if they had learned from friends, neither quantitative nor qualitative information is always being provided. This qualitative information is particularly important with regard to birth control. Experience will always be an important factor in learning about sex, and however much information is given, it can never prepare fully for the individual physical and emotional reactions.

But proper preparation for birth control use can make a
qualitative difference to early sexual experience. The
fact that half of the teenagers in this study said that
they were sexually experienced, and that many more would
become so before they married, means that teenage sex is
a 'fact of life'. It will not go away if we ignore it,
neither is it helpful to suggest that it should. In the
context of a society which encourages its members to care
for each other, sexual relationships may be said to be an
expression of that 'caring'. Early chapters demonstrated
that most young people believed in sex as part of a stable
and loving relationship. Most of the teenagers (86%) who
were having a sexual relationship with a member of the
opposite sex when they were interviewed had known their
partner for more than six months. Also, 88% of the girls
who were using the pill at the time of the interview had
been going out with their partners for over six months.
There is little evidence that young people regard abortion
as a method of contraception; in fact, the opposite would
seem to be true. Given this evidence, that most teenage
sexual relationships are not 'careless' or promiscuous,
society has a responsibility to ensure that it provides
birth control education at an age and of a kind which
will help young people to protect themselves from the
unwanted consequences of sexual intercourse.

SUMMARY

Most of the young people felt that lessons at school or
being told by parents was the best way to learn about
sex; over half mentioned lessons at school, and one in
three mentioned parents. Girls were more likely than
boys to mention parents in this context, and there were
divergent views on learning within a close family situation and a more formal school atmosphere.
     Less than a quarter of the teenagers were completely
satisfied with the way they themselves had learned about
sex. Critical evaluation of the way they had learned
suggested that they would have liked more detail about
reproduction, sexual intercourse and birth control at an
earlier age, and from what they regard as authoritative
sources.
     Those young people who had first learned about sex
from friends were more likely to be dissatisfied with the
way they had learned, and also more likely to be sexually
experienced.
     Birth control lessons at school increased knowledge
amongst those who were not sexually experienced. This,

together with the fact that young people thought lessons
at school were the best way to learn about birth control
and were more satisfied if they had learned in this way,
is a strong recommendation for birth control education in
schools.   This, in spite of the fact that there is no
obvious link yet between birth control lessons and use of
birth control.

14

CONCLUSIONS

The major concern of this study has been with and for
young people. In communities where they are growing up
with increasing freedom and mobility, and where they are
often exposed to conflicting influences, uncertainty
about the way to behave in personal relationships is an
almost inevitable consequence. As one girl said:
    'They should tell you how to behave when you go out
    with a boy, you know, what's right and wrong.'
This statement reveals uncertainty and a desire for
guidance, and also encompasses one of the main problems
for (sex) educators; that is, how to inform and guide
the young without increasing this uncertainty. In this
final chapter our findings are used as the basis for
discussion about ways in which young people may be
helped to make decisions about their own codes of
behaviour.

SEXUAL EXPERIENCE

Young people's attitudes to sex before marriage are in
line with what has been described as the 'widespread'
view in this country (International Planned Parenthood
Federation (Europe), 1975): approval in the context of a
stable and loving relationship, if care is taken to avoid
unwanted pregnancy. Half of the teenagers in this study
said they were sexually experienced, and although this may
be due to an increased willingness to say so, it does
reflect an increase in the numbers of teenagers who said
they were sexually experienced ten years ago. One in five
of all the young people said that their first experience
had been before they were 16. Boys were more likely to
say they were experienced than girls, and working-class
boys were more likely to have earlier experiences and

unprotected intercourse. Although teenage sexual activity
was not investigated in detail, there was little evidence
of promiscuity. The majority of young people currently
involved in a sexual relationship were having sex with
someone they had been going out with for more than six
months, and there was no evidence that the pill was
encouraging casual relationships, since most of the girls
who were taking the pill at the time of the interview had
known their partners for more than six months. Use of
birth control was widespread, only one in twelve of the
sexually experienced young people had never used any
method, and they were mainly boys. Although half of the
sexually experienced young people had sometimes taken a
chance and not used birth control, on the whole, use of
contraception showed a progression from the less reliable
methods to more effective ones. Even the girls who had
had abortions had been using birth control, albeit the
less reliable methods. This overall picture of teenage
use of birth control gives the lie to the image of careless and casual teenage sex often promoted by the media.
Although there are gaps in birth control use, particularly
at the initial stages of sexual experience, the majority
of teenagers held responsible attitudes to sex before
marriage. Given this evidence, two points should be made.
The media could often be more responsible in its presentation of teenage sexual behaviour than it is. When stories
of teenage pregnancy and abortion appear, some mention
should be made that they are atypical of the majority of
teenagers. Whilst details of such events make 'good
copy', if they are presented as frequent happenings,
teenagers themselves may believe it and suffer as a
result. One boy said during an interview:
    'I think I must be the only 18-year-old boy in the
    country who has not had sexual intercourse; it makes
    me feel bad.'
This kind of pressure can create unnecessary tension for
young people and could encourage them to have sex just
because they do not want to feel different.
    The second point, which is more important than the
alleviation of these kinds of public pressures, is the
need to provide adequate information about birth control
at relevant stages in adolescent development. Our
evidence suggests that young people want birth control
instruction in school and feel that lessons are a relevant
and appropriate source of information. It also suggests
that where lessons had been given they often presented
only generalised information, so that in 1974 only about
a fifth of young people were being told at school about
individual methods and how to use them. Some people would

not agree that lessons at school were the most appropriate
method of informing people about birth control, nor
teachers the best people to give that information.
Occasionally it did seem that teachers might be misinform-
ing their pupils. As far as we know, trainee teachers
are not given instruction in how to teach birth control,
which means that sex education teachers must rely on in-
service training or on their own knowledge of birth
control. There is a strong case for using specialist
teachers, doctors or para-medical workers for these kinds
of lessons. If they work closely with teachers there
should be few problems of continuity or lack of opportunity
for discussion after the information has been given. The
evidence on the use of outside speakers in sex education
suggests that it is successful and appreciated by young
people, and that in areas where lessons are carefully
prepared and followed up by teachers in the schools, pupil
satisfaction is increased.

METHODS OF BIRTH CONTROL

Because the pill is the most reliable method of birth
control available for young people, there has been a
tendency for its use to be promoted above other methods.
There are dangers in this promotion. First, girls may be
encouraged to take it when their pattern of sexual
activity does not warrant it. Although they may be
involved in stable relationships, because of their
circumstances, sexual intercourse may take place infrequently. Apart from the fact that many women do not
like the idea of introducing daily doses of drugs to
their systems, and that if a girl starts taking the pill
at sixteen she is faced with the possibility of taking
it for about 30 years, there is increasing evidence that
the pill reduces fertility (Vessey et al., 1976). Other
methods like the sheath, the cap and even the safe period,
if used properly, can be more satisfactory for irregular
or infrequent patterns of sexual activity. Full and
informed instruction on the use of the sheath and cap
with spermicides, and of how to use the safe period, would
enable girls and boys to use these methods effectively.
The IUD is also an alternative method which seems appropriate for teenagers, but is rarely mentioned as a
possibility for women who have not had children. This
may have been due to the risk of pelvic infection and low
toleration, but now that there is evidence that the pill
also carries risks, will teenagers be offered the IUD as
a real alternative? Although the pill is rightly

recommended for its reliability, one disadvantage of over-
selling it to teenagers is that it could discourage use
of other more appropriate methods.   There is a possibility
that boys could be discouraged from taking precautions
if they believe that every girl they meet is taking the
pill.

THE AGE OF CONSENT

The evidence on age of first experience suggests that one
in eight girls have at least one experience of sexual
intercourse before they are 16.   The numbers of girls at
risk of pregnancy at this early age is enough to merit
further consideration of changes in the law, if it can be
shown that such changes would encourage young people to
seek advice about, and use of, effective methods of birth
control.   The National Council for Civil Liberties, in a
report on sexual offences (1976), argues that the main
function of the law should be protective, and maintains
that 'the only reason for making sexual activity illegal
is because it may result in other people being harmed.
This rules out all laws concerned solely with morality.
It also rules out paternalistic laws which attempt to stop
an individual from harming himself; it is quite difficult
in reality, to harm oneself by having too much sex.'
These points seem valid, and if the evidence of doctors
working with young girls presents an accurate picture
and they are put off seeking advice on contraception
because they are under-age, then the law needs to be
adjusted so that its protective function can be maintained.

VENEREAL DISEASES

Statistics on the rising incidence of sexually transmitted
diseases amongst teenagers are sometimes used as an
indicator of increasing promiscuity.   The criteria on which
these statistics are reported vary from clinic to clinic,
and are currently the subject of an investigation (M. Adler,
private communication).   The figures which are used are
based on numbers of cases treated, so that some exaggera-
tion may occur.   Also, the proportion of the 16-19 age
group reported as having gonorrhea in 1974 was less than
half a per cent even though the incidence is increasing.
This is not to deny that venereal diseases are a cause for
concern, and any measures which can be taken to decrease
their prevalence are to be welcomed.   The evidence from
this study suggests that many young people are less than

well informed about the symptoms of these diseases. What
is more worrying is that nearly half of the teenagers who
thought they might have VD at some stage did nothing about
it. It seems likely that the shock treatment used by
parents and some teachers when information about VD is
being presented, has the opposite effect to the one
intended. If it is being used as a sanction against
sexual intercourse then the evidence suggests that it is
not working in that way, but simply encouraging fear and
hesitation when action may need to be taken. There is a
strong case for more balanced information about sexually
transmitted diseases which would allow those who did come
into contact with them to recognise the symptoms and to
take the necessary curative action.

USE OF BIRTH CONTROL SERVICES

On the whole, these young people seemed to have a good
idea about the availability of birth control services and
the advantages and disadvantages for them of using clinics
and general practitioners. The evidence suggests that
girls who had used the services were mostly satisfied
with their experiences. This may have been because their
expectations of the service were low. If this is so,
the problem becomes one of raising their expectations.
However, the current problem, if it can be seen as such,
is that the younger girls and most of the boys do not
use the services when or before they become sexually
experienced. There were few clues from them why this
was so, probably because we failed to ask enough or the
right questions. It could be that only those teenagers
who feel certain about their adult status use the services
and that others who might need them do not. Two possible
reasons for this are that the 'image' of clinics is such
that they are felt to be 'unavailable' by young girls and
the services they offer to be inappropriate for their
needs. If clinic use by young people is to be encouraged,
more emphasis should be placed on their advice-giving
function. There must be many teenagers who feel uncertain
about which method to use, even if they have extensive
knowledge of all the methods available. On the other hand,
the evidence from the study, that once girls decided to
seek advice, more of them chose their general practitioner,
could be an indication that extending clinic services for
young people is not the best way to meet their needs. The
case for specialised youth clinics could be argued, but we
feel uncertain about their value, partly because we did
not explore this question with the young people. Clinics

like the Brook Advisory Centre in London and Birmingham
obviously fulfil a need, but this is possibly because
their function is linked to pregnancy advice and abortion
services as well as birth control. An alternative
suggestion would be for a mobile counselling advisory
service to visit places where young people work and
gather in the evenings. This would have the advantage of
offering a range of skills to teenagers who might need
them, but would not see a birth control clinic as an
attractive or appropriate place to go.

There are two important advantages to this kind of
scheme: first, the service would be where the young
people are and would not involve them in journeys or
special efforts to make an appointment; second, the
service offers a range of skills. Advice about birth
control is not the only kind of advice young people want;
in fact, for most of them other problems are more pressing.
Relationships with parents, money, jobs, trouble with the
police, all these things and more can cause young people
to seek advice, and on many occasions, as we learned
during the interviews, just talking to an uninvolved adult
can be a help. Birth control advice should be offered as
part of a wider counselling service for young people, as
well as the specialised clinic and general practitioner
service which already exists. Counselling services do
exist, and it may be a question of supporting and
widening these rather than setting up a whole new network.
Most of them, however, have a 'specialised' image, and
it is this which can make young people feel that it is
not appropriate for them if they simply feel they want to
talk. There would be disadvantages to such a scheme - the
problem of waiting for the service to arrive is one. It
may be that the general practitioner service is a more
practical alternative. When we did this study, free
birth control advice had only just been introduced to
general practice, and it will be several years before we
can assess whether it is a relevant and workable system
for young people.

Birth control services have increased and improved
considerably during the past ten years, and these suggestions do not seek to undermine that achievement. The
falling incidence of abortion and premarital pregnancy
since 1974 are, in part, a testimonial to that achievement.
If they are to continue to increase their potential, gaps
in provision have to be identified. The gap which this
study has identified is that the younger sexually experienced girls, and boys, do not use the services. If they
were using methods which did not require service provision,
this would not matter, but the evidence suggests that they

do not always do this and accidents occur. Information
and advice are a necessary preliminary to birth control
use. Some of this can be provided through lessons at
school, but at some stage most individuals who are sexually
experienced or about to become so might feel the need for
specialist advice. It is then that the availability and
accessibility of services becomes important. The fact
that teenage boys do not use the services is not necessarily a bad sign. The sheath is the method used most
frequently by them, and this does not need to involve
clinic or general practitioner visits. Machines in pubs
were the most common place of purchase (39% of sheath
users had bought their supplies from this place). A case
could be made for expanding outlets of this kind, but
they do not have the advantage of ensuring careful use of
the sheath. It is obvious that boys will not need to use
clinics and doctors in the same way that girls do, since
all the reversible medical methods of contraception are
female methods. There is no real need for them to use
the services for supplies, but if the services were to
extend their advice-giving role, then young men might be
encouraged to use them. One other point about male use
of services might be made. Sexual activity involves male
and female, and there were hints from some girls that the
weight of responsibility for contraception lay too
heavily upon women. This is inevitable because the more
reliable methods are female methods; and also of course
it is the girl who gets pregnant. But the responsibility
for avoiding pregnancy should be a shared one, even if
the methods used are female. The women's movement is
making some progress in helping women to question whether
it is right for the emphasis to be on female use of
methods, and many couples do, in fact, share the responsibility. However, at the early stages of a relationship,
discussions about which method to use could be difficult
and embarrassing, and it is at this stage that service
providers could encourage both partners to attend. Some
girls indicated that they felt happier and more confident
attending clinics when their boyfriends went with them.
Encouraging male use of services might fulfil two
functions: that of helping boys to share in the responsibility for birth control use, and of encouraging girls to
use the services.

One of the major findings of this and other similar
studies was the different emphasis given to the sex education of boys and girls. If services could encourage and
help boys to become more responsible and better informed,
a step would be taken to redress the present imbalance.

LEARNING ABOUT SEX

Three important findings emerged from the examination of
sources of information about sex and birth control which
merit further discussion. First, that there is no clear
causal relationship between early information sources and
teenage sexual behaviour. Given the lengthy and complex
nature of the learning process, we did not expect to be
able to say that there was. Some patterns did emerge,
however, which are worthy of attention. Both boys and
girls who had first learned about sex from friends were
more likely to be sexually experienced. They were also
more likely to say that they were dissatisfied with the
way that they had learned. Although a causal relationship
is not established, we might speculate that inadequate
information about sex could lead young people to experiment
and 'find out for themselves'. On the other hand, friends
were often regarded as a useful and important source at
later stages of the learning process. Reconciliation of
these two stages of need in the learning process is
important, and it must be said that it was the teenagers
themselves who identified these two stages for us. When
they were asked what they thought the best way to learn
about sex was, many of them named an authoritative source
like school or parent as the first source, and then went
on to say that afterwards discussion with friends or
'someone who knows' was part of the best way to learn.
The dissatisfaction with friends as a first source of
information and the greater satisfaction expressed if
school or parents had been the first source, emphasises
the need for information to be provided by adults at an
early enough stage so that young people can feel confident
that they know the 'facts' and can use them as a basis for
fuller discussions with friends and other adults. Friends
can be important for discussions of information and
emotions; this role should not be undermined by their
being the first source of information. If it is, then the
chances of young people feeling uncertain about the
information they have received from this source are high.
If parents and schools can see the necessity of providing
information at an early enough stage, so that young
people's need for information to come from what they
regard as the best and authoritative sources can be
fulfilled, uncertainty might be reduced and satisfaction
increased.

PARENTS AND SCHOOLS

The parents interviewed in this study did feel that they
should be involved in telling their children about
reproduction and sexual intercourse, but a minority had
actually told them or discussed the subject. Where
information had been given, mothers assumed a greater
responsibility than fathers, who seemed to support this
with their beliefs about sources of information, and by
allowing mothers to 'do' most of the telling. The gap
between their beliefs and their actions is crucial in
understanding the past inadequacies of sex education.
Because parents believe they should be the ones to tell
their children about sex, schools have been reluctant
to begin their sex education lessons before parents have
had a chance to raise the subject. While both parents
and schools hesitate, the information which children seek
is passed to them from friends. There are difficulties
in suggesting remedies for this situation. From the
findings, it is clear that many young people and their
parents see lessons at school as the best way to learn
about sex. The logical recommendation would be, therefore,
that children should have lessons in basic reproduction
in primary school at a fairly early age. This might
stimulate them to ask their parents questions, and the
parents, from our evidence, would find it easier to
respond than to initiate discussions. Parents' fears and
uncertainties about giving information at too early a
stage, risking the destruction of 'innocence', could be
allayed. The raising of the subject by children would be
enough to allow some parents to discuss sex freely - other
parents might still find it difficult, and a few might
never feel able to. Primary and secondary schools might
help these parents by inviting them to come to previews
of the lessons. In this way, parents could be informed
of what their sons and daughters would be learning, which
might help uncertain parents to enter into discussions
with them.

It was inevitable that this study would end with a plea
for improving sex education in schools because, as Gagnon
and Simon point out (1973, p.21), schools are the one
source of information which are accessible to change.
Although we feel that there are many schools which could
improve the quality and quantity of sex education, we are
not unaware of the problems involved. Reproduction and
birth control are difficult subjects to teach. Children
will laugh and fool about to cover their embarrassment or
difficulties with the subject. A teacher needs to be sure
of her ground before she stands up in front of a class of

30 teenage boys and girls to describe how to use the
sheath. There will always be some parents who object to
sex education lessons, and head teachers will be faced
with the problems of meeting their objections. It may
be that visiting doctors and outside speakers would be
more effective at some stages, whereas other earlier
stages would benefit from one teacher following through a
series of lessons. These kinds of details are best worked
out by educators. What this study has done is to point
out that those young people who had first learned about
sex at school were more likely to be satisfied with the
way they had learned than those who had first learned
from friends; that over half of them thought that school
was the best way to learn about sex and birth control;
and that if they had had lessons on birth control, their
knowledge of how to use individual methods was greater
than those who had not had lessons. These findings should
encourage those already working in the field of sex
education, and stimulate those schools where very little
sex education is taught to include it in the curriculum.

METHODS AND RESPONSE

SAMPLE SOURCE

Once the decision had been taken to limit the target
population to the 16-19 age group, four sources were
considered for the selection of the young people: school
registers, executive council lists, local authority
rating lists and the electoral register. In practice,
after some consideration, only the electoral register
was tested as a sampling frame in the pilot study.

School registers These were rejected primarily because
they could only have given a sample of under-17s, when
the target sample was the 16-19 age group. In theory,
this source could have given a sample of the 13-15 age
group but, as Schofield (1965, pp.17 and 277) discovered,
some education authorities refuse permission for their
registers to be used for this purpose. In addition, the
Department of Education and Science had informed the
Institute, through the Department of Health, that they
did not wish the schools to be used for the study.

The executive council lists Permission to use these
lists has to be sought from each executive council, and
some councils have been known to refuse. But primarily
this list was rejected because the reorganisation of the
Health Service in April 1974 meant that lists were not
likely to be available in time.

The rating list These lists can provide an up-to-date
and accurate list of dwellings but there are three major
disadvantages. It is not possible from the list alone to
locate households within dwellings. A written approach
would have to be addressed to 'the occupier' rather than
a named resident. Also, the lists, although up-to-date,

are often difficult to use because of corrections and additions. But finally, local authority reorganisation made it unlikely that these lists would be available in a usable form.

The electoral register   This aims to list the names and addresses of all British subjects resident in the UK on the qualifying date who are, or will become, 18 during the life of the register. The register, which is based on information gathered in the autumn, is published the following February and effective for one year. However, it has been demonstrated by Gray and Gee (1967, p.13) that voters who have moved since the autumn will be wrongly recorded (3% by date of publication and 11% by the end of the life of the register), and some potential voters will be excluded completely (about 4%) either through mis-understandings about eligibility (e.g. by Commonwealth citizens and young people) or because they move so often that they never register at all.

The registers are probably more complete as a frame of addresses than of individuals, since the exclusion of a person will cause their address to be omitted only if the same happens to all other persons resident there. New addresses occupied after the autumn, and addresses with no eligible voters resident, are clearly excluded completely. In some unpublished Social and Community Planning Research work (mentioned in Technical Manual No.2, 1972, p.41) in four London polling districts, between 6% and 17% of addresses were missing. These districts were, however, especially likely to have omissions, and the true omission rate is probably much lower.

Moreover, the use of electoral registers as a sampling frame in the pilot study demonstrated that a representa-tive sample of 16-19-year-olds could be found in this way.

SELECTION OF YOUNG PEOPLE

The young people for the study were located by writing to a random sample of addresses from the electoral register in 12 areas in England and Wales, explaining the purpose of the study and asking if anyone aged 16-19 lived at that address.

The areas

The areas were chosen with probability proportional to

their populations by use of a sampling fraction on the
cumulative population of a listing of the new local
authority districts grouped within their counties. The
counties were listed in order from north to south to give
an appropriate spread over the country. The areas finally
selected had the boundaries of the new local authority
districts. Twelve areas were chosen because it seemed
the minimum number to give the sample a claim to be
nationally representative, and the largest number that
could be practically administered in terms of interviewer
teams. Also because it would yield a suitable number of
completed interviews in each area to allow regional
analysis. The areas chosen were:

Tyne & Wear (b)   Tynemouth C.B.; Wallsend M.B.; Whitley
   Bay M.B. (part); Longbenton U.D.; Seaton Valley U.D.
   (part). Pop.207,000.
Humberside (1)   Bridlington M.B.; Driffield U.D.;
   Bridlington R.D. (part); Driffield R.D.; Pocklington
   R.D. Pop. 65,434.
Merseyside (d)   Huyton with Roby U.D.; Kirkby U.D.;
   Prescot U.D.; Whiston R.D. (part); West Lancashire
   R.D. (part). Pop.198,000.
South Yorkshire (c)   Sheffield C.B.; Stocksbridge U.D.;
   Wortley R.D. (part). Pop.566,000.
Salop (3)   Shrewsbury M.B.; Atcham R.D. Pop. 82,329.
West Midlands (e)   Birmingham C.B.; Sutton Coldfield
   M.B. Pop. 1,096,000.
Gloucestershire (5) Cirencester U.D.; Cirencester R.D.;
   North Cotswold R.D.; Northleach R.D.; Tetbury R.D.
   Pop. 62,765.
Mid-Glamorgan (1) Bridgend U.D.; Maesteg U.D.; Ogmore &
   Garw U.D.; Porthcawl U.D.; Penybont R.D. Pop.123,414.
London Croydon. Pop.333,840.
London Redbridge. Pop.239,880.
Kent (4) Gillingham M.B. Pop. 86,714.
Devon (5) Ashburton U.D.; Buckfastleigh U.D.; Dawlish
   U.D.; Newton Abbott U.D.; Teignmouth U.D.; Newton
   Abbott R.D.; St Thomas's R.D. (that part not in
   district 7). Pop. 91,793.
The decision to use the new Metropolitan and non-
Metropolitan districts was taken to allow comparison with
future studies.

Sample size

Deciding how many addresses need be approached to obtain
a completed sample of about 1,400 young people involved
some complicated calculations. It was possible to

calculate from Census data how many young people a given
number of households should yield, and pilot study results
also gave information about this and response rates to the
type of approach to be used. It was thus possible to
predict that the completed sample size would be 7% of the
total number of addresses approached. To produce a
completed sample of 1,400 it was therefore necessary to
write to approximately 19,000 addresses. Equal numbers
of addresses were selected from the electoral registers
in each of the 12 areas (since areas had already been
chosen with probability proportional to population). Thus
any area variations in numbers of young people per household were reflected in the sample. Because addresses were
being selected and not individuals, the procedure known
as 'firsting' was used to give each address an equal
chance of being selected (see Social and Community
Planning Research, 1972, p.42, for details). A total of
19,224 addresses were written to to find out whether
anyone aged 16-19 lived at that address.

THE POSTAL SCREEN

The letters

Although addresses and not individuals were selected from
the electoral registers, the letter was addressed to an
individual at that address. It used to be thought that
postal questionnaires were inadequate for screening
purposes because of the low response rates achieved. But
in recent years a number of postal surveys have achieved
high response rates (Scott, 1961). It is also known that
the sponsorship and the length of the questionnaire
affect the response rate (Moser and Kalton, 1971,
pp.262-3). With these considerations in mind, a letter
was drafted containing only essential information; to
this was attached a form with two questions. The aim was
to minimise time and effort for the respondent in an
attempt to get the largest possible response rate. The
letter and questionnaire were as follows:
    I am writing to ask for your help with a study we are
    doing about young people and the health and education
    services. We would like to know whether you or anyone
    at your address is aged 16, 17, 18 or 19. Please count
    anyone of that age who lives at your address, even if
    they are not part of your family and even if they are
    married.

    We would also like to know if anyone of that age

normally lives there, but is studying or working away
from home.

Please could you answer the two questions on the
attached form and return it to us straight away in the
stamped envelope provided. Just two ticks are needed.
Even if there is no-one of that age living there we
would still like to know this.

You may like to know that the Institute for Social
Studies in Medical Care is a non-profit making research
organisation. We have written a number of books and
articles about the health and welfare services.

Your name and address was chosen from the list of
voters in your area.

Thank you for your help,

                    Yours sincerely

                    Christine Farrell

                                        CONFIDENTIAL

Young people and health and education services

PLEASE PUT A TICK (√) BESIDE YOUR ANSWERS TO THE
QUESTIONS

1. Is there anyone aged 16, 17, 18 or 19 living at
    your address?

                    Yes - male   _____

                    Yes - female   _____

                    Yes - male and female   _____

                    No-one aged 16, 17,
                    18 or 19   _____

2. Is there anyone aged 16, 17, 18 or 19 who normally
    lives at your address but is living or working
    away from home at the present time?

                    Yes - male   _____

                    Yes - female   _____

Yes - male and female   _____

No-one aged 16, 17,
18 or 19   _____

PLEASE RETURN THIS FORM STRAIGHT AWAY IN THE PREPAID
ADDRESSED ENVELOPE PROVIDED. THANK YOU FOR YOUR HELP.

After two weeks, those who had not replied were sent the
following reminder letter:

About a week ago, I wrote to a number of people,
including yourself, asking whether there is anyone
aged 16, 17, 18 or 19 living at your address.

Most of the people have now replied, but I have not
heard from you. It would be a great help if you could
return the completed form, as soon as possible.

If you have already replied, we are sorry to have
troubled you unnecessarily.

Thank you for your help.

Yours sincerely,

Christine Farrell

After a further four weeks a second reminder letter was
sent to those who had still not replied:

About a fortnight ago I wrote to you asking for your
help with our study about young people and the health
and education services. As I have not yet heard from
you, I expect the form never reached you or has got
mislaid, so I am sending you another form with a prepaid addressed envelope.

I hope you will be able to spare a moment to send it
off. If you have already replied, we are sorry to have
troubled you unnecessarily.

Yours sincerely,

Christine Farrell

Originally the intention had been to post the second
reminder two weeks after the first reminder, but the
response was so low that mailing was postponed for a
further two weeks. One reason for this was the postal
go-slow which delayed delivery and returns. Another
reason which we began to suspect after examining the
response to the first letter was the type of reply
envelope enclosed. Other Institute studies (e.g.
Cartwright, 1964) using the same type of postal approach,
and our own pilot study, had shown a pattern of response
after each mailing stage which suggested that something
was going wrong with the response at this point. Table
A1 shows that pattern compared with what happened at the
first and second stage of this survey.

TABLE A1   Pattern of response to the postal screen
compared with the pilot study and another Institute study

	Previous Institute study	Pilot study	Main study
Reply after 1st letter	60%	58%	39%
Reply after 1st reminder	17%	15%	14%
Reply after 2nd reminder	15%	16%	27%
Overall response	92%	89%	80%

The only difference in this study which was likely to
account for the lower response rate at the first stage
was the business reply envelope which had been enclosed
for return of the form. In the pilot study an ordinary
stamped envelope had been used, and it seemed possible
that the official, business looking envelope was
encouraging people not to reply. A business reply
envelope is easily thrown away because it does not waste
a stamp - to throw away an envelope which is already
stamped does seem much more wasteful. For the second
reminder a stamped addressed envelope was substituted for
the business reply envelope, and the response rate
increased.

The response

Table 1 in the Introduction shows that 77.7% replied to
this letter, 1.2% wrote or indicated that they were

refusing to reply, O.9% of the addresses no longer existed
(house demolished), and 20.2% did not respond. All the
letters returned marked 'gone away, address unknown' were
returned addressed to the occupier. The total number of
gone aways was 488, and of these 337 remained unanswered.
The 151 who did reply are included in the totals in Table
A1.

Stages of response

It might be expected, in this kind of postal screen, that
the people giving a positive reply (i.e. those who had
young people aged 16-19 living at their address) would
be more or less reluctant to reply than those providing
a negative reply. In this case there is some evidence
to suggest that they were slightly more reluctant, and
that more of them replied at the second and third stages
of the screen. Table A2 shows that the proportion of
positive replies was greater after the first and second
reminders than it was after the first letter.

TABLE A2   Type of reply and stage received

	After 1st letter	After 1st reminder	After 2nd reminder	All replies
	%	%	%	%
Replied				
Had young person aged 16-19	11.0	13.5	12.6	12.0
Had no young person aged 16-19	88.1	83.3	82.5	85.4
Total replied	99.1	96.8	95.1	97.4
Wrote refusing to answer	O.2	1.5	3.4	1.5
Informed house void/occ.dead	0.7	1.7	1.5	1.1
Number of replies (= 100%)	7,483	2,719	5,138	15,340

TABLE A3 Response by area

	Tyne & Wear side %	Humber side %	Mersey side %	South Yorks. %	Mid-Glam. %	Salop. %	W.Mid-lands %	Glouc/shire %	Croy-don %	Red-bridge %	Kent %	Devon %	All areas %
Replied	80.0	82.0	72.3	81.0	80.7	78.7	73.8	78.9	72.7	75.9	78.1	78.5	77.7
Refused	1.0	1.4	0.9	0.8	0.6	1.2	0.8	1.5	1.3	1.4	1.5	1.8	1.2
House void/ dead	0.9	0.9	1.3	1.6	0.2	1.3	1.2	0.9	0.3	0.6	0.6	1.0	0.9
No response	18.1	15.7	25.5	16.6	18.5	18.8	24.2	18.7	25.7	22.1	19.8	18.7	20.2
No.written to (=100%)	1,602	1,602	1,602	1,602	1,602	1,602	1,602	1,602	1,602	1,602	1,602	1,602	19,224

TABLE A4 Response from northern and southern areas

	Northern areas %	Midland areas %	Southern areas %	All areas %
Replied	78.8	78.1	76.3	77.7
Refused	1.0	1.0	1.5	1.2
House void/dead	1.2	0.9	0.6	0.9
No response	19.0	20.0	21.6	20.2
Number written to (= 100%)	6,408	6,408	6,408	19,224

Northern areas: Tyne & Wear; Humberside; South Yorkshire and Merseyside.
Midland areas: Salop; West Midlands; Gloucestershire; Mid-Glamorgan.
Southern areas: Croydon; Redbridge; Kent; Devon.

Response by area

The reply rate within the 12 areas varied from the highest, 82.0% in Humberside, to the lowest, 72.3% in Merseyside. On the whole the reply rate was lower from the large industrial areas and highest in the rural areas. There was very little difference in the rate of reply between northern and midland regions, but the southern region produced a slightly lower reply rate than the other two regions. Tables A3, A4 and A5 show the response rate in each area and the differential rate of response between northern, midland and southern areas, and Metropolitan and non-Metropolitan districts.

TABLE A5   Response from Metropolitan and non-Metropolitan districts

	Metropolitan districts	Non-Metropolitan districts	All areas
	%	%	%
Replied	75.9	79.5	77.7
Refused	1.0	1.3	1.2
House void/dead	1.0	0.8	0.9
No response	22.1	18.4	20.2
Number written to (= 100%)	9,612	9,612	19,224

Metropolitan districts:	Tyne & Wear; Merseyside; South Yorkshire; West Midlands; Croydon; Redbridge.
Non-Metropolitan districts:	Humberside; Salop; Mid-Glamorgan; Gloucestershire; Kent; Devon.

One explanation for the different response rate in Metropolitan and non-Metropolitan districts could be that more of the people we wrote to had moved, since mobility is greater in industrial areas. Another possible explanation is that people in Metropolitan districts are more often approached in this way for help with market research and other kinds of research, and for this reason may be less likely to respond.

The problems of non-response

The reply rate of 78% is lower than the rate achieved in the pilot study (82%) and lower than that achieved in other studies of this type. For example, a reply rate of 87% was reached in 'Human Relations and Hospital Care' (Cartwright, 1964), and Scott (1961) reports response rates of around 90% in five Government surveys. Since the non-response represents a fifth of the total sample, we considered taking some action either to increase the response rate or to approach a sample of non-respondents in order to attempt to assess the nature of the bias.

The possible courses of action were:

(a) To increase the response rate by sending out a fourth letter

This would have involved sending out 3,884 letters. The cost in time and money would have been high - over £1,000 - and the reply rate might well have been as low as 15% - which would add only 3% to the overall reply rate. Added to this, these people have already resisted answering three letters, and would probably feel (rightly) that they were being badgered. The original 80% reply rate had given a total of 1,840 addresses where 16-19-year-olds lived - and as the refusal rate for interviews on the pilot was not inordinately high, there was no need to increase the actual *size* of the sample, since we originally aimed at a completed sample of around 1,400. During the postal survey we received over 200 angry telephone calls and letters from people who threatened to take 'further action' if they were bothered again. These people was promised that they would not be approached again.

It seemed sensible, therefore, to conclude that the likely improvement in the level of the reply rate would not justify the necessary expenditure of time and money or the possible damage to the Institute's reputation.

(b) To explore the nature of the possible bias amongst the group of non-respondents

This could have been done in two ways: by post, or by sending interviewers to call at a sample of non-responding addresses:

(i) A postal survey to a sample of non-respondents would have most of the disadvantages outlined under (a), except that it would have been cheaper. In addition, to find out anything at all about the nature of non-responders, we should have needed to enclose a questionnaire. The chances of them completing and returning a longer, more personal form, when they have already failed to return a form asking only two questions, seemed remote.

(ii) A call on a random sample of 10% of the non-responders would have involved 33 addresses in each area. Because the original sample was not clustered,

some of these addresses could have been as much as 20
miles apart. Paying interviewers time and travel costs
would have run into hundreds of pounds. There was the
additional problem of exposing interviewers to angry
members of the public, and a risk of some kind of public
outcry against the Institute.
Although the reply rate to the postal screen is not as
high as we would have liked, the question which really
needed to be asked was: will the final outcome of the study
be impaired if no action is taken either to increase the
reply rate or to calculate the nature of the possible bias
amongst non-responders? Although we would have liked to
attempt to improve this situation, it seemed that the disadvantages involved in any attempt to improve the results
outweighed the possible gains. The important thing would
seem to be to have a final sample with characteristics as
near to the national figures as possible.

Testing the validity of the 'no' responders

A further methodological problem in postal surveys is the
validity of the answers received from those people giving
negative replies. Again we considered approaching a
sample of those who had replied saying that no young
people aged 16-19 lived at the address, but similar
disadvantages applied. Costs, already high, would have
increased disproportionately, and the more serious
ethical problem of appearing to badger and disbelieve
respondents led to a decision not to attempt this.
  Against these problems of response to the postal
screen, there is one compensating factor. The size of
the final sample of 16-19-year-olds produced from the
1,840 positive replies was greater than had been predicted
by the pilot study. Seven per cent of 19,224 initial
letters should have given a completed sample of 1,346;
in fact, it was 1,556.

INTERVIEW RESPONSE RATE

Once the young people had been found, the more serious
problems of co-operation had to be faced. Had it been
possible to approach the young people directly, some of
the problems of parental interference might have been
avoided. As it was, we had no names or indications of
relationships, so that it was not possible to ask to
speak to 'Guy Fawkes' or 'your son' or 'your lodger'. Nor
was it possible to write them a personal letter explaining

what we wanted, as Schofield did in his study.   In a sense
we had to face a double chance of refusal.   The risk of
either parent refusing to allow their child to participate
was one of the reasons why it was decided to interview a
sample of mothers and fathers at the same time.

Interviewers were given the full name and address of
the named person and instructed to ask to speak to this
person.   They were then to remind him about his reply to
the Institute which indicated that one or more 16-19-year-
old lived at this address.   This was usually readily
recalled.   This person was then asked to supply, for all
young people in the age group, name, date of birth,
relationship to the named person and, if temporarily away
from home, their other address and details of when they
would be returning.   If the named person was in the age
group the interviewer was to proceed with an explanation
of the aim of the study - that the study was of the
interests and attitudes of young people to school, work
and the health services, and particularly how young people
learn about reproduction, sex and birth control, both at
school and elsewhere - and wherever possible to complete
the interview immediately.   When this was not convenient
an appointment was made.   The young person was to be told
that the interview would take about an hour.

Where the named person was not a young person aged
16-19, the interviewer had to ask to speak to him.   At
this stage it was often necessary to give the parent
(usually the named person) some explanation of the study
before it was possible to see the young person.   The
explanation to the parent was less full, and referred more
to health education and reproduction than to sex and birth
control.

Refusals

Altogether, 346 young people refused to take part in the
study (16% of 2,110 approached).   Neither the difference
in the proportions of boys and girls refusing (17% compared
with 16%) nor the difference in the numbers of boys and
girls approached for interview (1,078 compared with 1,032)
was significant.   Table A7 shows the types of refusals and
the comparative proportions of males and females refusing.
This table indicates that girls were more likely than boys
to refuse for themselves.   The girls were also more likely
to refuse for themselves than to have a parent refuse for
them.   There is no significant difference between proportions of girls (31%) and boys (36%) having a parent refuse
for them.   This is an unexpected finding, because it seemed

TABLE A6   Response to interview approach by area

	Tyne & Wear side	Humber side	Mersey side	South Yorks.	Mid-Glam.	Salop.	W.Mid-lands	Glouc/shire	Croy-don	Red-bridge	Kent	Devon	All areas
	%	%	%	%	%	%	%	%	%	%	%	%	%
Completed interviews	74	78	81	73	78	72	75	78	76	67	65	64	74
Refusals	18	12	15	20	10	14	15	12	15	24	17	26	16
Not available for interview	8	10	4	7	12	14	10	10	9	9	18	10	10
No. of young people (= 100%)	188	161	221	168	183	190	190	183	159	164	155	148	2,110
No. of addresses approached	163	135	184	154	164	173	159	151	138	154	136	129	1,840

A7   Type of refusal by sex

Type of refusal	Male	Female	All refusals
	%	%	%
Direct refusal by young person	29	40	34
Direct parental refusal before young person seen	36	31	34
Indirect refusals: never in, appointments broken etc.	35	29	32
Number (= 100%)	179	167	346

likely that parents might be more protective of girls than boys, especially in the light of figures from Schofield's study, where 26% of girls' refusals came from the parents compared with 17% of the boys' (Schofield's overall refusal rate was 15%). The fact that parental refusals formed a larger proportion in this study than in Schofield's may be explained by the fact that Schofield was able to write his initial approach letter directly to the teenagers, and thus bypass some parental objections.

Analysis of the response to interview by area, using the same broad areas as in Table A4, revealed that northern and midland areas had less refusals than the southern area. The northern area had correspondingly fewer young people who were unavailable for interview. There are a number of possible explanations for these differences. Southerners may co-operate more reluctantly because they are approached to help with surveys more often than northerners, who, added to this, may be less mobile than those in southern areas.

An attempt was made to collect some information about the age and social class (by father's occupation) of the young people who refused. This was often a difficult task, and although interviewers were briefed to collect this information, the person refusing was not always prepared to give it. Consequently, the proportion of people who gave information about age and social class was low. Response to the question about age varied from 32% in one area to 90% in another, and response to the question about social class was, in one area, as low as 4%, and 26% averaged over all the areas. No valid analysis of the characteristics of the people who refused was possible.

Ten per cent of the sample of young people approached were unavailable for interview (10% of boys, 9% of girls). More than 208 were initially classified as unavailable, and whenever possible these people were followed up and interviews attempted. However, many of them were living outside the study areas and the cost of obtaining these interviews would have been too high to allow an approach to all.

The interview response rate of 74%, although not as high as some other Institute studies, seems reasonable for a study involving such a highly mobile and unpredictable group.

THE INTERVIEWERS

Normally the practical considerations of recruiting men

and training them swings the argument in favour of using
female interviewers, but because we had to recruit young
people, most of them without interviewing experience, we
felt justified in recruiting male and female interviewers.
Two male and two female interviewers worked in each of the
twelve areas, the males interviewing boys and fathers, and
the females interviewing girls and mothers. We did not
feel it was advisable to switch interviewers on a sample
of interviews, and are therefore not in a position to test
whether the sex of the interviewer affected the response
rate. The only possible indication we have is that the
response rate is higher than it was on the pilot study
(74% compared with 72%) when female interviewers were
used to interview males and females. But this could be
due to a range of factors, and is in no way clear evidence
that the sex of the interviewer affected the response rate.
It was not possible to calculate the differential male and
female response rate for the pilot study, because at that
stage we did not always know the sex of the non-responders.
In the main study, 72% of all males were interviewed and
75% of all females.

THE TEENAGERS

Apart from the following details about the proportions of
young people in each age group who were still at school,
the characteristics of the sample have been described
fully in the Introduction. From Table A8 it is clear
that the biggest difference between the sample and the
total population is amongst the 16-year-olds. It is
possible that this difference arose because the DES
figures were gathered in the January of 1974, and must
have included some 16-year-olds who had left school by
the time of the interview period (July 1974 to February
1975). (It should be noted that the figures in Table A8
are not directly comparable, since the DES figures cover
the whole of the United Kingdom, whereas the sample was
drawn from England and Wales.)

TABLE A8 Comparison with national figures* of proportions
who are still at school in each age group

	All UK	Sample population	
	% of age group still at school	% of age group still at school	Total numbers in each age group (= 100%)
16	45.5%	38.7%	351
17	20.3%	22.5%	404
18+	6.9%	1.9%	801

*Department of Education and Science actual age distribu-
tions of school pupils in January 1974, published in
Social Trends 1975 (table 8.2).

INITIAL APPROACH SHEET

1...........Eldest young person

2...........2nd young person

3...........Mother

4...........Father

5...........Other young person

INITIAL APPROACH SHEET:
Young People's Knowledge of Birth Control
Summer 1974

INTRODUCTION: I'm from the Institute for Social Studies
in Medical Care in London. We wrote to this address a
few weeks ago to ask if anyone aged 16, 17, 18 or 19
lived here. Mr (M/S) _____ was kind enough to write
back to say that there was. Could you tell me if a young
person of that age:

		Yes	No
	1. lives here with you?	1	2
ASK ALL FOUR	2. lives at this address but in another household?	1	2
	3. normally lives at this address but is living away at the moment?	1	2
	4. has moved since we wrote to this address in May?	1	2

FOR EACH CATEGORY CODED GO THROUGH ALL APPROPRIATE STAGES.

STAGE 1   FOR THOSE WHERE YOUNG PERSON LIVES IN THE HOUSE-
          HOLD INITIALLY APPROACHED. 'We are writing a
          book about young people, the jobs they do, the
          way they spend their free time and their educa-
          tion. We are particularly interested in the
          health education they had at school. (We also
          want to talk to their mothers and fathers.)
          Could you tell me how many young people aged 16,
          17, 18 or 19, live with you; their name(s), age,
          when they were born; and if they are related to
          you?' FILL IN THESE DETAILS ON THE FORM ON THE
          BACK OF THIS SHEET FOR ALL 16, 17, 18 OR 19 YEAR
          OLDS. THEN SAY: 'Could I speak to him/her?'
          IF YOUNG PERSON IS OUT: FIND OUT WHEN THEY WILL
          BE IN AND ARRANGE TO CALL BACK. IF YOUNG PERSON
          IS IN AND YOU SPEAK TO HIM/HER - REPEAT STAGE
          1 'We are writing a book ...' and say 'Could I
          talk to you now? The interview takes about 50
          minutes ....' IF NOT CONVENIENT MAKE AN APPOINT-
          MENT FOR AS SOON AS POSSIBLE.

STAGE 2   FOR THOSE LIVING AT THIS ADDRESS BUT IN A
          DIFFERENT HOUSEHOLD SAY: 'I'd like to talk to
          him/her, could you tell me his/her name and
          when he/she is likely to be in?' THANK PERSON
          FOR HELP AND TRY TO CONTACT YOUNG PERSON. WHEN
          FOUND CARRY OUT STAGE 1. RECORD NAME AND ANY
          OTHER DETAILS OBTAINED ON TABLE 1 OVER.

STAGE 3   FOR THOSE WHERE YOUNG PERSON IS WORKING OR
          STUDYING AWAY FROM HOME - SAY: 'We are writing
          a book about young people, the jobs they do, the
          way they spend their free time and their educa-
          tion. Could you tell me how many young people
          aged 16, 17, 18 or 19 usually live here; their
          name(s), age, when they were born; and if they
          are related to you?' FILL THESE DETAILS IN FORM
          ON THE BACK. THEN SAY: 'Could you say when he/
          she is likely to be at home?' ASK FOR ADDRESS
          OF YOUNG PERSON LIVING AWAY FROM HOME AND WRITE
          IN FORM ON BACK PAGE. IF YOUNG PERSON WILL BE
          AT HOME DURING THE NEXT TWO MONTHS TRY TO
          ARRANGE AN APPOINTMENT.

MOTHER OR FATHER INTERVIEWS. ALL THIS APPLIES IF MOTHER
          OR FATHER INTERVIEWS ARE REQUIRED. BUT, IN
          ADDITION AT STAGE 1 YOU MUST EXPLAIN THAT YOU
          WANT TO INTERVIEW MOTHER/FATHER AT THE SAME TIME.
          'We would also like to ask Mothers/Fathers what

they think about these things. Could I arrange
a time when it would be convenient to talk to
both you and your son/daughter (mother/father)?'
MAKE APPOINTMENT AND EXPLAIN THAT YOU WILL BRING
A COLLEAGUE WHO WILL INTERVIEW THE YOUNG PERSON
SEPARATELY.

STAGE 4   IF NAMED PEOPLE HAVE MOVED AWAY - ASK WHERE THEY
HAVE GONE. RECORD NEW ADDRESS IN RECORD OF CALLS.
ASK IF ANYONE AGED 16, 17, 18 OR 19 LIVES THERE
NOW. CARRY ON WITH STAGE 1.

IF EITHER YOUNG PERSON OR MOTHER/FATHER REFUSE
AFTER ALL EFFORTS, TRY TO FIND OUT WHY, WITH:

1.   Could you say why you don't want to take part
     in the study?

2.   Could you say why you don't want your son/
     daughter to help with the study?

3.   Would you mind telling me what job you (IF
     FATHER), your husband (IF MOTHER), your
     father does?

4.   And could you just tell me who lives here
     besides yourself?

INTERVIEWER'S COMMENTS.

OUTCOME
PLEASE CODE ALL THAT APPLY

1. Number of young people eligible for interview.

    None 0
    One 1
    Two 2
    Three 3
    Four 4

2. Number of young people interviewed.

    None 0
    One 1
    Two 2
    Three 3
    Four 4

3. Mother to be interviewed.

IF YES   Yes 1
(1)   No 2
          Interviewed 3
          Not interviewed.. 4

4. Father to be interviewed.

IF YES   Yes 1
(1)   No 2
          Interviewed 3
          Not interviewed.. 4

IF FAILED TO GET ANY INTERVIEW COMPLETE NEXT SECTION.

5. FAILURE RECORD
    Reason for not doing interview:

	young person	mother	father
Direct refusal for self	1	1	1
Inconvenient and appointments not kept	2	2	2
Never in	3	3	3
Moved and can't trace	4	4	4
Not available for interview (e.g. at sea, in prison)	5	5	5
Left the country	6	6	6
Wrong information - no young person here	7	7	7

5.   FAILURE RECORD (Contd)

	young person	mother	father
Original addresses untraceable	8	8	8
No mother/no father	9	-	-
Not living with parents at all	-	9	9
Any other circumstances (describe)..	O	O	O

_____

_____

IF DIRECT OR INDIRECT REFUSAL (1) or (2)
(a) Person refusing was:

	young person	mother	father
Young person	1	1	1
Mother	2	2	2
Father	3	3	3
Husband	4	4	4
Wife	5	5	5
Someone else (specify).............	6	6	6

6.   Interviewer's assessment of failure.
     Describe what happened.

TABLE 1   DETAILS OF YOUNG PEOPLE AT THIS ADDRESS OR LIVING AWAY FROM HOME.

Name	M F	Date of Birth	Relationship to informant	Address if living away from home
	M F			
	M F			
	M F			
	M F			

RECORD OF CALLS

Date	Time	Outcome	Who seen

RECORD NEW ADDRESSES BELOW

Appointment made for: Date   Time

Interviewer's number _____   Number of colleague doing parent interview _____

METHODS USED FOR SELECTING
AND INTERVIEWING PARENTS

SAMPLE OF PARENTS

The sample of parents was drawn from the 1,840 positive
replies to the postal screen described in Appendix I.
One in every three of these addresses was randomly
selected for parent and young people interviews. Once
this sample of 601 had been drawn, alternate addresses
were allocated to either the mother or father of eligible
young people.

TABLE A9   Sample of addresses for parent and young people
interviews

	Mothers	Fathers	Total
Number of addresses in main sample	-	-	1,840
Number of addresses selected for parent interview (1 in 3)	301	300	601
Exclusions because wrong information from postal screen (no young people lived there)	13	23	36
Total remaining addresses where a parent interview attempted	288	277	565

The natural parent was to be interviewed, and the only
'substitute' parents eligible were adopting parents, step-
parents, or permanent foster parents where the natural

parent no longer featured in the young person's life. In
the event, 4% of those parents interviewed were substitute
parents (10 step-parents, 5 adoptive).

THE INTERVIEW

The approach at those addresses where a parent was to be
seen was necessarily more complicated than those where
only the young people were to be interviewed. An appointment usually had to be made because the parent and young
person were to be interviewed simultaneously, but by
different interviewers. The preliminaries and explanations happened in two stages.

First stage - initial approach

In addition to the procedure already described (Appendix
I) for approaching the young people, the interviewer had
to explain that the mother or father was also included in
the study, by saying: 'We would also like to ask mothers/
fathers what they think about these things.' There were
then three instructions which influenced and complicated
the arrangements to be made. For reasons of confidentiality and confidence, the interviewer used for the parents
was always different from those who interviewed the young
people in the family. To avoid collaboration between
members of the same family, the interviews were to be
carried out at the same time. Finally, separate rooms
were essential to avoid inhibiting eavesdropping. In
spite of these inconveniences to the family, 62% of
parents and 86% of the young people co-operated. The
need for privacy and confidentiality was generally
appreciated. Because appointments were usually made for
these interviews, opportunities for discussion between
parent and young person did occur. To minimise this
possibility the interviewer kept preliminary explanations
about the nature and aims of the study as unspecific as
possible. Although there is no evidence of discussions
affecting outcome, it seems likely that any inclination
to co-operate or refuse was reinforced during this
interval. There is evidence that parental refusals and
young person refusals were linked, since only 33% of young
people whose parents refused agreed to be interviewed,
compared with 87% of those whose parents also agreed.
Amongst all the young people whose parents were approached
for interview, the proportion refusing was 21% compared
with 14% of those young people whose parents were not
approached for interview.

Second stage - the appointment

The second part of these preliminaries took place when
the interviewers returned, as arranged, to complete the
interviews. It was usually unnecessary to repeat the
earlier introduction, but at this stage both informants
were assured of confidentiality. The following introduction was made to parents, and the interviewer offered to
answer any questions about the study:

'Shall I tell you a bit more about the study? We are
talking to 1,500 young people all over the country,
about their interests, jobs and about their secondary
education. We are particularly interested in the kind
of health education lessons they had in school. We
are talking to parents because we feel it is important
to know how they feel about their children's interests
and education and particularly what young people should
be told about sex and birth control. Anything you tell
us will be treated as confidential, we don't use any
names or identify anyone at all in the reports we
write. Some of the questions are fairly personal, but
if you don't want to answer a particular question just
say so.'

When the parent had been satisfied on all these points,
he or she was asked for details of family composition
and dates of birth of children. From this information
it was possible to check that all eligible 16-19-year-olds
had been located and approached. It was also at this
point that the interviewer could establish for those
parents who had more than one child in the age group which
young person was to be the focus of the subsequent
questions. It had been decided that parents would be
asked for their views in relation to boys only or girls
only, as it was possible that they would hold different
views on sex education for girls and boys. Interviewers
selected this 'key' child as follows: where there was
only one young person in the age group there was no
problem, he or she was the 'key' child about whom parents
were questioned. Where there were two or four young
people aged 16-19, the elder was selected if the family
serial number ended in an odd number, the younger where
it ended in an even number. The middle child was chosen
where there were three in the age group. In the event
of there being five eligible young people, the interviewer
was instructed to choose the eldest child if the serial
number ended in an even number, the youngest if it were
an odd number.

Duration of interview and interruptions

Most interviews (68%) took between 45 and 90 minutes.
None took less than 30 minutes, and a few (7%) took two
hours or more. Interruptions were few. Only 6% had what
the interviewer recorded as 'many' interruptions. Almost
two-thirds (62%) were entirely free from intrusions. For
the remaining 20%, a husband or wife was the person most
likely to have been present.

RESPONSE RATE

The parents' interview response rate (62%) is lower than
the rate for the young people (74%). More parents than
young people refused (25% compared with 16%) but similar
numbers of parents and young people were unavailable for
interview (13% compared with 10% of young people). The
refusal rate for mothers and fathers was almost the same,
as were the proportions of mothers and fathers unavailable
for interview.

It is possible that the parents' response rate is lower
than the young people's because of the way the interviewers
were briefed. They were told that priority should be
given to the interviews with young people. If it seemed
likely that they might lose a teenage interview by
persisting with an unwilling parent, they should stop
trying to arrange the joint interview and simply interview the young person. In addition, interviewers were
selected primarily on an assessment of their ability to
relate to young people. This is not to say that their
skill in handling parents was disregarded, but their
comparative youthfulness may have been off-putting for
some parents.

Reasons for refusals and unavailability

One in four (144) of the parents approached for interview
refused. The reasons they gave for refusing were
analysed, and over a third (37%) said that they had no
time to spare or were not interested in the study.
Others (31%) were more direct and said that they felt
their privacy was being invaded, that they felt they had
been deceived by the postal screening or that they
objected to the subject of the study. Another 15%
refused to give a reason, and a small group (7%) broke
appointments or otherwise evaded the interviewers. In
10% of the families approached, sickness or family trouble
was given as a reason for refusing.

Of the parents who were unavailable for interview
(72), half (51%) lived out of the area and could not be
reached during the interviewing period. This group
included fathers away at sea, parents of foreign young
people, and separated parents. A quarter of them (25%)
had moved away and proved untraceable. Dead or very sick
parents accounted for another fifth (21%). The remaining
3% were unavailable for reasons which could not be classified in any of these groups.

PARENTAL CHARACTERISTICS

The interviewers were asked to get minimal information
about refusing or unavailable parents (e.g. father's
occupation and family composition), but for obvious
reasons they were not always successful. So few of those
who refused were prepared to state their own or their
husband's occupation that the social class of the non-
responders is not known. However, when asked about family
composition, particularly children in the 16-19 age group,
the refusing informants were more prepared to give
information. Taken in conjunction with replies to the
postal screening, this information leads us to believe
that the non-responding parents had similar numbers of
children aged 16-19 to the parents who agreed to take
part. Table A10 shows that there is no significant
difference between average numbers of young people per
parent in each of the parent categories. An average of
1.2 young people aged 16.19 was also typical of the
families of the larger sample of young people.

TABLE A10 Number of 16-19-year-olds in families of
co-operating and non-co-operating parents

Parental category	Number of parents	Number of children aged 16-19	Average per parent
Interviewed parents	349	425	1.2
Refusing parents	144	180	1.3
Unavailable parents	72	86	1.2
Totals	565	691	1.2

POSSIBLE BIAS AMONGST INTERVIEWED PARENTS

More mothers (186) than fathers (163) were interviewed,
although the difference is not significant. These 349
parents had a total of 1,093 children of all ages, an
average of 3.1 per parent/family. The interviewed
mothers had more children in their families (an average
of 3.3) than interviewed fathers (average 2.9). Since
parents were not asked for their age or date of marriage,
we cannot compare their family size with other studies.
However, because couples without children were obviously
not included, one would expect the average number of
children per parent to be greater than the national
average. There is also likely to be a bias towards those
with larger families, as those with more children have a
greater chance of having at least one aged 16-19 years.
    Parents were asked for the father's current or most
recent occupation; fathers therefore reported for themselves and mothers for the fathers. Table A11 shows the
social class distribution. Mothers were more likely not
to give a classifiable occupation for the father, and the
social class distribution of the mothers' families leans
less towards the middle class than the fathers'. It is
possible that working-class fathers were less willing to
be interviewed or less available than middle-class
fathers, perhaps because of longer working hours and
shift hours.

TABLE A11 Social class (by father's occupation) of
mothers and fathers by sex of key child

	MOTHERS		FATHERS		All parents
	Male	Female	Male	Female	
	%	%	%	%	%
Middle class	36	35	48	45	41
Working class	55	56	48	51	53
Unclassified	9	9	4	4	6
Number = 100%	95	91	89	74	349

    Between them the 349 parents had 425 children aged
16-19 years, and of these, 53% were boys and 47% were
girls. The differences in numbers of boys and girls is
not significant. The parents were asked for their
opinions in relation to a particular child. The selection
procedure described earlier led to the distribution of
male and female parents and young people illustrated in
Table A12.

TABLE A12   Sex of parent interviewed by sex of 'key' child

	Boys	Girls	Totals
Mothers	26%	27%	53%
Fathers	26%	21%	47%
Totals	52% (180)	48% (169)	100% (349)

Of these 349 'key' children, 88% were interviewed, thus making possible in 307 cases a detailed comparison of the parental and adolescent views of sex education and of interaction in the particular family. An additional 60 children of these parents were interviewed, but since the parents were not asked for their views and recollections in relation to these particular young people, they cannot be included in the group of joint studies.

FAMILY COMPOSITION

Almost two-thirds (63%) of the parents had mixed sex families. Of the remainder, equal numbers had all boys or all girls in their families (21% and 16%). Almost one-third (31%) of the 'key' children were eldest children. One-seventh (14%) were only children, and the rest were in the middle, or the youngest child in the family (55%). Most of the 'key' children (88%) lived at home with their parents.

SELF-ADMINISTERED QUESTIONNAIRE
FOR YOUNG PEOPLE   SUMMER 1974

Serial Number
_____

Could you tick (√) what you think is the answer to these questions or statements about some methods of contraception. Please only tick (√) one answer to each question.

1. Two questions about the sheath (french letter, Durex, johnny)

    a) If a boy is using the sheath when should he put it on his penis?

	It makes no difference when	_____ 1
ONLY	An hour before intercourse	_____ 2
TICK	After he has reached climax (come off)	_____ 3
ONE	Immediately before entering the	
ANSWER	girl's vagina	_____ 4
	Really don't know	_____ 5
	Don't understand	_____ 6

    b) If you or your partner use a sheath are you:

ONLY	More likely to get VD	_____ 1
TICK	Less likely to get VD	_____ 2
ONE	It doesn't make any difference	_____ 3
ANSWER	Really don't know	_____ 4
	Don't understand	_____ 5

2. Two questions about the pill

    (a) When a girl first goes on the pill is she protected from pregnancy immediately?

Yes	....	_____ 1
No	....	_____ 2
Really don't know	....	_____ 3
Don't understand	....	_____ 4

b)   There is a serious risk of getting pregnant if a
     girl forgets to take the pill for more than:

     12 hours .... _____ 1
     24 hours .... _____ 2
     36 hours .... _____ 3
     48 hours .... _____ 4
     Really don't know .... _____ 5
     Don't understand .... _____ 6

3. One question about withdrawal (taking care)
     If the boy pulls his penis out of the girl
     before he reaches a climax (comes off) she is
     less likely to get pregnant.

ONLY   True   .... _____ 1
TICK   False   .... _____ 2
ONE   Really don't know .... _____ 3
ANSWER   Don't understand .... _____ 4

4. One question about the 'safe' period (rhythm method)
     At what time in a girl's monthly cycle is she
     most likely to get pregnant.

          Just before her periods .... _____ 1
ONLY   Just after her periods   .... _____ 2
TICK   Middle (between periods) .... _____ 3
ONE   Any time .... _____ 4
ANSWER   Really don't know .... _____ 5
          Don't understand .... _____ 6

5. One question about the IUD (coil, loop, copper seven)
     An IUD can only be fitted for someone who has
     had at least one pregnancy.

ONLY   True   .... _____ 1
TICK   False   .... _____ 2
ONE   Really don't know .... _____ 3
ANSWER   Don't understand .... _____ 4

6. One question about foams, jellies, creams, C-film
     What is the correct way to use chemical methods
     such as foams, creams, jellies, tablets, c-films?

ONLY   Absolutely on their own .... _____ 1
TICK   With sheath/or cap   .... _____ 2
ONE   Really don't know   .... _____ 3
ANSWER   Don't understand   .... _____ 4

7. And one about VD
        You can get VD:

ONLY	Only from someone of the opposite sex	_____	1
TICK	From someone of either sex	_____	2
ONE	Really don't know	_____	3
ANSWER	Don't understand	_____	4

BIBLIOGRAPHY

BELL, N.W. and VOGEL, E.F. (1961), 'A Modern Introduction to the Family', London, Routledge & Kegan Paul.
BELSON, W.A. (1975), 'Juvenile Theft: The causal factors', London, Harper & Row.
BERNSTEIN, B. (1971), 'Class, Codes and Control', London, Routledge & Kegan Paul.
BONE, M. (1973), 'Family Planning Services in England and Wales', London, HMSO.
BOTT, E. (1957), 'Family and Social Network', London, Tavistock.
CARTWRIGHT, A. (1964), 'Human Relations and Hospital Care', London, Routledge & Kegan Paul.
CARTWRIGHT, A. (1967), 'Patients and their Doctors', London, Routledge & Kegan Paul.
CARTWRIGHT, A. (1970), 'Parents and Family Planning Services', London, Routledge & Kegan Paul.
CARTWRIGHT, A. (1976), 'How Many Children?', London, Routledge & Kegan Paul.
CARTWRIGHT, A. and LUCAS, S. (1974), Survey of Abortion Patients for the Committee on the working of the Abortion Act, 'Report of the Committee on the Working of the Abortion Act', vol.III, London, HMSO.
CARTWRIGHT, A. and MOFFETT, J. (1974), A Comparison of Results Obtained by Men and Women Interviewers in a Fertility Survey, 'Journal of Biosocial Science', vol.6, pp.315-22.
CENTRAL STATISTICAL OFFICE (1974), 'Social Trends 1974', London, HMSO.
CENTRAL STATISTICAL OFFICE (1975), 'Social Trends 1975', London, HMSO.
COSER, R.L. (ed.) (1974), 'The Family, its Structures and Functions', London, Macmillan.
CROW, D. (1971), 'The Victorian Woman', London, Allen & Unwin.

DALLAS, D. (1972), 'Sex Education in School and Society', National Foundation for Education Research.

DAVIES, J. and STACEY, B. (1972), 'Teenagers and Alcohol', London, HMSO.

DEPARTMENT OF EDUCATION AND SCIENCE (1975), 'Statistics of Education, 1974', vol.I, Schools, HMSO.

DEPARTMENT OF HEALTH AND SOCIAL SECURITY (1975), 'Health and Personal Social Services Statistics for England', London, HMSO.

DEPARTMENT OF HEALTH AND SOCIAL SECURITY (1975), 'Health and Personal Social Services Statistics for Wales', London, HMSO.

DOUGLAS, J.W.B. (1964), 'The Home and the School', London, MacGibbon & Kee.

DOUGLAS, J.W.B. (1966), The age of reaching puberty, 'The Scientific Basis of Medicine Annual Review', pp.91-105.

FOGELMAN, K. (ed.) (1976), 'Britain's Sixteen-Year-Olds', London, National Children's Bureau.

GAGNON, J.H. and SIMON, W. (1973), 'Sexual Conduct', London, Hutchinson.

GILL, D.G., ILLESLY, R. and KOPLIK, L.H. (1970), Pregnancy in teenage girls, 'Social Science and Medicine', vol.3, pp.549-74.

GILL, D.G., REID, G.D.B. and SMITH, D.M. (1974) Sex Education: Press and parental perceptions' in ROGERS, R.S. (ed.) 'Sex Education, Rationale and Reaction', London, Cambridge University Press.

GRAY, P.G. and GEE, F.A. (1967) 'Electoral Registration for Parliamentary Elections', London, HMSO.

HARGREAVES, D.H. (1967), 'Social Relations in a Secondary School', London, Routledge & Kegan Paul.

HARGREAVES, D.H. (1972), 'Interpersonal Relations and Education', London, Routledge & Kegan Paul.

HARRIS, A. (1974), What Does Sex Education Mean? in ROGERS, R.S. (ed.) 'Sex Education, Rationale and Reaction', London, Cambridge University Press.

HOGGART, R. (1957), 'The Uses of Literacy', London, Chatto & Windus.

HUTCHINSON, F.D. (1976), The Effect of the Law Regarding the Age of Consent, 'The Journal of Family Planning Doctors', vol.1, no.4, pp.10-11.

ILLSLEY, R. and TAYLOR, R. (1974), Sociological Aspects of Teenage Pregnancy, unpublished report for the World Health Organisation.

INTERNATIONAL PLANNED PARENTHOOD FEDERATION (EUROPE) (1975), 'A Survey on the Status of Sex Education in European Member Countries', London, IPPF.

KANTNER, J.F. and ZELNIK, M. (1972a), The Probability of Premarital Intercourse, 'Social Science Research', vol.1, no.3, pp.335-41.

KANTNER, J.F. and ZELNIK, M. (1972b), Sexual Experience of Young Unmarried Women in the United States, 'Family Planning Perspectives', vol.4, no.4.

LEESON, J. and STEIN, Z. (1964), Approaching the Menarche, 'The Medical Officer', 12.6.64, pp.342-4.

McCANCE, C. and HALL, D.J. (1972), Sexual Behaviour and Contraceptive Practice of Unmarried Female Undergraduates at Aberdeen University, 'British Medical Journal, vol.2, pp.694-700.

MECHANIC, D. (1968), General Practice in England and Wales, 'Medical Care', vol.6, no.3.

MORGAN, D.H.J. (1975), 'Social Theory and the Family', London, Routledge & Kegan Paul.

MOSER, C.A. and KALTON, G. (1971), 'Survey Methods in Social Investigation', London, Heinemann Educational Books.

MUSGROVE, F. (1964), 'Youth and the Social Order', London, Routledge & Kegan Paul.

NATIONAL COUNCIL FOR CIVIL LIBERTIES (1976), 'Sexual Offences', evidence to the Criminal Law Revision Committee, NCCL Report No.13, London, National Council for Civil Liberties.

NEWSON, J. and E. (1968), 'Four Years Old in an Urban Community', London, Allen & Unwin.

NIEMI, R.G. (1974), 'How Family Members Perceive Each Other', London, Yale University Press.

OFFICE OF POPULATION CENSUSES AND SURVEYS (SOCIAL SURVEY DIVISION) (1973), 'General Household Survey 1973', London, HMSO.

OFFICE OF POPULATION CENSUSES AND SURVEYS (1975), 'Population Trends 2', London, HMSO.

OFFICE OF POPULATION CENSUSES AND SURVEYS (1975), 'Population Trends 1', London, HMSO.

OSOFSKY, H.J. (1971), Adolescent Sexual Behaviour: Current status and anticipated trends for the future, 'Clinical Obstetrics and Gynaecology', 14, pp.393-408.

PARSONS, T. and BALES, R.F. (1955), 'Family, Socialisation and Interaction Process', Chicago, Free Press.

PEARCE, D. (1975), Births and Family Formation Patterns, 'Population Trends 1', London, HMSO, pp.6-8.

PLUMMER, K. (1975), 'Sexual Stigma', London, Routledge & Kegan Paul.

RAINWATER, L. (1965), 'Family Design: Marital sexuality, family size, and contraception', Chicago, Aldine Publishing Co.

REISS, I.L. (1970), Premarital Sex as Deviant Behaviour, 'American Sociological Review', vol.35, no.1, pp.78-87.

REISS, I.L. (1971), 'The Family System in America', New York, Holt, Rinehart & Winston.

264   Bibliography

ROBERTS, D.F. and DANN, T.C. (1975), A 12-year Study of
Menarchealage, 'British Journal of Preventive and Social
Medicine', vol.29, pp.31-9.
SCHOFIELD, M. (1965), 'The Sexual Behaviour of Young
People', London, Longmans.
SCOTT, C. (1961), Research on Mail Surveys, 'Journal of
Royal Statistical Society', Series A, vol.124, pp.143-205.
SEYMOUR-SMITH, M. (1975), 'Sex and Society', London,
Hodder & Stoughton.
SIREY, E.C. and POWER, M.J. (1974), 'Tower Hamlets
Household Survey', Clearing House for Local Authority
Social Services: University of Birmingham.
SOCIAL AND COMMUNITY PLANNING RESEARCH (1972), 'Sample
Design and Selection', Technical Manual 2, London, SCPR.
SORENSON, R.C. (1973), 'Adolescent Sexuality in Contem-
porary America', New York, World Publishing Co.
THOMPSON, J. (1976), Fertility and Abortion Inside and
Outside Marriage, 'Population Trends 5', London, HMSO,
pp.3-8.
VENNER, A.M. (1972), The Sexual Behaviour of Adolescents
in Middle America, 'Marriage and the Family 34', pp.696-
705.
VESSEY, M., DOLL, R., PETO, R., JOHNSON, B. and WIGGINS, P.
(1976), A Long-Term Follow-up Study of Women using
Different Methods of Contraception: An interim report,
'Journal of Biosocial Science', vol.8, no.4.
WILLMOTT, P. (1966), 'Adolescent Boys of East London',
London, Routledge & Kegan Paul.

INDEX

Routledge Social Science Series

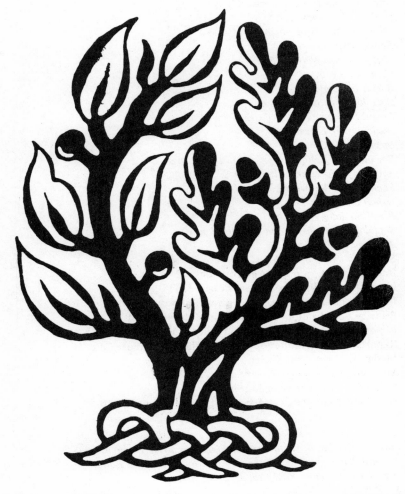

Routledge & Kegan Paul   London, Henley and Boston

39 Store Street, London WC1E 7DD
Broadway House, Newtown Road, Henley-on-Thames,
Oxon RG9 1EN
9 Park Street, Boston, Mass. 02108

Contents

Authors wishing to submit manuscripts for any series in
this catalogue should send them to the Social Science Editor,
Routledge & Kegan Paul Ltd, 39 Store Street,
London WC1E 7DD

●*Books so marked are available in paperback*
All books are in Metric Demy 8vo format (216 × 138mm approx.)

International Library of Sociology

General Editor John Rex

GENERAL SOCIOLOGY

Barnsley, J. H. The Social Reality of Ethics. *464 pp.*
Belshaw, Cyril. The Conditions of Social Performance. *An Exploratory Theory. 144 pp.*
Brown, Robert. Explanation in Social Science. *208 pp.*
● Rules and Laws in Sociology. *192 pp.*
Bruford, W. H. Chekhov and His Russia. *A Sociological Study. 244 pp.*
Cain, Maureen E. Society and the Policeman's Role. *326 pp.*
●**Fletcher, Colin.** Beneath the Surface. *An Account of Three Styles of Sociological Research. 221 pp.*
Gibson, Quentin. The Logic of Social Enquiry. *240 pp.*
Glucksmann, M. Structuralist Analysis in Contemporary Social Thought. *212 pp.*
Gurvitch, Georges. Sociology of Law. *Preface by Roscoe Pound. 264 pp.*
Hodge, H. A. Wilhelm Dilthey. *An Introduction. 184 pp.*
Homans, George C. Sentiments and Activities. *336 pp.*
Johnson, Harry M. Sociology: *a Systematic Introduction. Foreword by · Robert K. Merton. 710 pp.*
●**Keat, Russell,** and **Urry, John.** Social Theory as Science. *278 pp.*
Mannheim, Karl. Essays on Sociology and Social Psychology. *Edited by Paul Keckskemeti. With Editorial Note by Adolph Lowe. 344 pp.*
  Systematic Sociology: *An Introduction to the Study of Society. Edited by J. S. Erös and Professor W. A. C. Stewart. 220 pp.*
Martindale, Don. The Nature and Types of Sociological Theory. *292 pp.*
●**Maus, Heinz.** A Short History of Sociology. *234 pp.*
Mey, Harald. Field-Theory. *A Study of its Application in the Social Sciences. 352 pp.*
Myrdal, Gunnar. Value in Social Theory: *A Collection of Essays on Methodology. Edited by Paul Streeten. 332 pp.*
Ogburn, William F., and **Nimkoff, Meyer F.** A Handbook of Sociology. *Preface by Karl Mannheim. 656 pp. 46 figures. 35 tables.*
Parsons, Talcott, and **Smelser, Neil J.** Economy and Society: *A Study in the Integration of Economic and Social Theory. 362 pp.*
Podgórecki, Adam. Practical Social Sciences. *About 200 pp.*
●**Rex, John.** Key Problems of Sociological Theory. *220 pp.*
  Sociology and the Demystification of the Modern World. *282 pp.*
●**Rex, John** (Ed.) Approaches to Sociology. *Contributions by Peter Abell, Frank Bechhofer, Basil Bernstein, Ronald Fletcher, David Frisby, Miriam Glucksmann, Peter Lassman, Herminio Martins, John Rex, Roland Robertson, John Westergaard and Jock Young. 302 pp.*
Rigby, A. Alternative Realities. *352 pp.*
Roche, M. Phenomenology, Language and the Social Sciences. *374 pp.*

Sahay, A. Sociological Analysis. *220 pp.*

Simirenko, Alex (Ed.) Soviet Sociology. *Historical Antecedents and Current Appraisals. Introduction by Alex Simirenko. 376 pp.*

Strasser, Hermann. The Normative Structure of Sociology. *Conservative and Emancipatory Themes in Social Thought. About 340 pp.*

Urry, John. Reference Groups and the Theory of Revolution. *244 pp.*

Weinberg, E. Development of Sociology in the Soviet Union. *173 pp.*

FOREIGN CLASSICS OF SOCIOLOGY

●**Durkheim, Emile.** Suicide. *A Study in Sociology. Edited and with an Introduction by George Simpson. 404 pp.*

●**Gerth, H. H.,** and **Mills, C. Wright.** From Max Weber: *Essays in Sociology. 502 pp.*

●**Tönnies, Ferdinand.** Community and Association. *(Gemeinschaft und Gesellschaft.) Translated and Supplemented by Charles P. Loomis. Foreword by Pitirim A. Sorokin. 334 pp.*

SOCIAL STRUCTURE

Andreski, Stanislav. Military Organization and Society. *Foreword by Professor A. R. Radcliffe-Brown. 226 pp. 1 folder.*

Carlton, Eric. Ideology and Social Order. *Preface by Professor Philip Abrahams. About 320 pp.*

Coontz, Sydney H. Population Theories and the Economic Interpretation. *202 pp.*

Coser, Lewis. The Functions of Social Conflict. *204 pp.*

Dickie-Clark, H. F. Marginal Situation: *A Sociological Study of a Coloured Group. 240 pp. 11 tables.*

Glaser, Barney, and **Strauss, Anselm L.** Status Passage. *A Formal Theory. 208 pp.*

Glass, D. V. (Ed.) Social Mobility in Britain. *Contributions by J. Berent, T. Bottomore, R. C. Chambers, J. Floud, D. V. Glass, J. R. Hall, H. T. Himmelweit, R. K. Kelsall, F. M. Martin, C. A. Moser, R. Mukherjee, and W. Ziegel. 420 pp.*

Johnstone, Frederick A. Class, Race and Gold. *A Study of Class Relations and Racial Discrimination in South Africa. 312 pp.*

Jones, Garth N. Planned Organizational Change: *An Exploratory Study Using an Empirical Approach. 268 pp.*

Kelsall, R. K. Higher Civil Servants in Britain: *From 1870 to the Present Day. 268 pp. 31 tables.*

König, René. The Community. *232 pp. Illustrated.*

●**Lawton, Denis.** Social Class, Language and Education. *192 pp.*

McLeish, John. The Theory of Social Change: *Four Views Considered. 128 pp.*

Marsh, David C. The Changing Social Structure of England and Wales, *1871-1961. 288 pp.*

Menzies, Ken. Talcott Parsons and the Social Image of Man. *About 208 pp.*

Mouzelis, Nicos. Organization and Bureaucracy. *An Analysis of Modern Theories. 240 pp.*

Mulkay, M. J. Functionalism, Exchange and Theoretical Strategy. *272 pp.*

Ossowski, Stanislaw. Class Structure in the Social Consciousness. *210 pp.*

Podgórecki, Adam. Law and Society. *302 pp.*

Renner, Karl. Institutions of Private Law and Their Social Functions. *Edited, with an Introduction and Notes, by O. Kahn-Freud. Translated by Agnes Schwarzschild. 316 pp.*

SOCIOLOGY AND POLITICS

Acton, T. A. Gypsy Politics and Social Change. *316 pp.*

Clegg, Stuart. Power, Rule and Domination. *A Critical and Empirical Understanding of Power in Sociological Theory and Organisational Life. About 300 pp.*

Hechter, Michael. Internal Colonialism. *The Celtic Fringe in British National Development, 1536–1966. 361 pp.*

Hertz, Frederick. Nationality in History and Politics: *A Psychology and Sociology of National Sentiment and Nationalism. 432 pp.*

Kornhauser, William. The Politics of Mass Society. *272 pp. 20 tables.*

Kroes, R. Soldiers and Students. *A Study of Right- and Left-wing Students. 174 pp.*

Laidler, Harry W. History of Socialism. *Social-Economic Movements: An Historical and Comparative Survey of Socialism, Communism, Co-operation, Utopianism; and other Systems of Reform and Reconstruction. 992 pp.*

Lasswell, H. D. Analysis of Political Behaviour. *324 pp.*

Martin, David A. Pacifism: *an Historical and Sociological Study. 262 pp.*

Martin, Roderick. Sociology of Power. *About 272 pp.*

Myrdal, Gunnar. The Political Element in the Development of Economic Theory. *Translated from the German by Paul Streeten. 282 pp.*

Wilson, H. T. The American Ideology. *Science, Technology and Organization of Modes of Rationality. About 280 pp.*

Wootton, Graham. Workers, Unions and the State. *188 pp.*

CRIMINOLOGY

Ancel, Marc. Social Defence: *A Modern Approach to Criminal Problems. Foreword by Leon Radzinowicz. 240 pp.*

Cain, Maureen E. Society and the Policeman's Role. *326 pp.*

Cloward, Richard A., and **Ohlin, Lloyd E.** Delinquency and Opportunity: *A Theory of Delinquent Gangs. 248 pp.*

Downes, David M. The Delinquent Solution. *A Study in Subcultural Theory. 296 pp.*

Dunlop, A. B., and **McCabe, S.** Young Men in Detention Centres. *192 pp.*

Friedlander, Kate. The Psycho-Analytical Approach to Juvenile Delinquency: *Theory, Case Studies, Treatment. 320 pp.*

Glueck, Sheldon, and **Eleanor.** Family Environment and Delinquency. *With the statistical assistance of Rose W. Kneznek. 340 pp.*

Lopez-Rey, Manuel. Crime. *An Analytical Appraisal. 288 pp.*

Mannheim, Hermann. Comparative Criminology: *a Text Book. Two volumes. 442 pp. and 380 pp.*

Morris, Terence. The Criminal Area: *A Study in Social Ecology. Foreword by Hermann Mannheim. 232 pp. 25 tables. 4 maps.*

Rock, Paul. Making People Pay. *338 pp.*

●**Taylor, Ian, Walton, Paul,** and **Young, Jock.** The New Criminology. *For a Social Theory of Deviance. 325 pp.*

●**Taylor, Ian, Walton, Paul,** and **Young, Jock** (Eds). Critical Criminology. *268 pp.*

SOCIAL PSYCHOLOGY

Bagley, Christopher. The Social Psychology of the Epileptic Child. *320 pp.*

Barbu, Zevedei. Problems of Historical Psychology. *248 pp.*

Blackburn, Julian. Psychology and the Social Pattern. *184 pp.*

●**Brittan, Arthur.** Meanings and Situations. *224 pp.*

Carroll, J. Break-Out from the Crystal Palace. *200 pp.*

●**Fleming, C. M.** Adolescence: Its Social Psychology. *With an Introduction to recent findings from the fields of Anthropology, Physiology, Medicine, Psychometrics and Sociometry. 288 pp.*

● The Social Psychology of Education: *An Introduction and Guide to Its Study. 136 pp.*

●**Homans, George C.** The Human Group. *Foreword by Bernard DeVoto. Introduction by Robert K. Merton. 526 pp.*

● Social Behaviour: *its Elementary Forms. 416 pp.*

●**Klein, Josephine.** The Study of Groups. *226 pp. 31 figures. 5 tables.*

Linton, Ralph. The Cultural Background of Personality. *132 pp.*

●**Mayo, Elton.** The Social Problems of an Industrial Civilization. *With an appendix on the Political Problem. 180 pp.*

Ottaway, A. K. C. Learning Through Group Experience. *176 pp.*

Plummer, Ken. Sexual Stigma. *An Interactionist Account. 254 pp.*

●**Rose, Arnold M.** (Ed.) Human Behaviour and Social Processes: *an Interactionist Approach. Contributions by Arnold M. Rose, Ralph H. Turner, Anselm Strauss, Everett C. Hughes, E. Franklin Frazier, Howard S. Becker, et al. 696 pp.*

Smelser, Neil J. Theory of Collective Behaviour. *448 pp.*

Stephenson, Geoffrey M. The Development of Conscience. *128 pp.*

Young, Kimball. Handbook of Social Psychology. *658 pp. 16 figures. 10 tables.*

SOCIOLOGY OF THE FAMILY

Banks, J. A. Prosperity and Parenthood: *A Study of Family Planning among The Victorian Middle Classes. 262 pp.*

Bell, Colin R. Middle Class Families: *Social and Geographical Mobility. 224 pp.*

6

Burton, Lindy. Vulnerable Children. *272 pp.*
Gavron, Hannah. The Captive Wife: *Conflicts of Household Mothers.*
190 pp.
George, Victor, and **Wilding, Paul.** Motherless Families. *248 pp.*
Klein, Josephine. Samples from English Cultures.
   1. Three Preliminary Studies and Aspects of Adult Life in England.
   447 pp.
   2. Child-Rearing Practices and Index. *247 pp.*
Klein, Viola. The Feminine Character. *History of an Ideology. 244 pp.*
McWhinnie, Alexina M. Adopted Children. *How They Grow Up. 304 pp.*
● **Morgan, D. H. J.** Social Theory and the Family. *About 320 pp.*
● **Myrdal, Alva,** and **Klein, Viola.** Women's Two Roles: *Home and Work.*
238 pp. 27 tables.
Parsons, Talcott, and **Bales, Robert F.** Family: Socialization and Inter-
action Process. *In collaboration with James Olds, Morris Zelditch and
Philip E. Slater. 456 pp. 50 figures and tables.*

SOCIAL SERVICES

Bastide, Roger. The Sociology of Mental Disorder. *Translated from the
French by Jean McNeil. 260 pp.*
Carlebach, Julius. Caring For Children in Trouble. *266 pp.*
George, Victor. Foster Care. *Theory and Practice. 234 pp.*
   Social Security: *Beveridge and After. 258 pp.*
George, V., and **Wilding, P.** Motherless Families. *248 pp.*
● **Goetschius, George W.** Working with Community Groups. *256 pp.*
Goetschius, George W., and **Tash, Joan.** Working with Unattached Youth.
416 pp.
Hall, M. P., and **Howes, I. V.** The Church in Social Work. *A Study of
Moral Welfare Work undertaken by the Church of England. 320 pp.*
Heywood, Jean S. Children in Care: *the Development of the Service for the
Deprived Child. 264 pp.*
Hoenig, J., and **Hamilton, Marian W.** The De-Segregation of the Mentally
Ill. *284 pp.*
Jones, Kathleen. Mental Health and Social Policy, 1845-1959. *264 pp.*
King, Roy D., Raynes, Norma V., and **Tizard, Jack.** Patterns of Residential
Care. *356 pp.*
Leigh, John. Young People and Leisure. *256 pp.*
● **Mays, John.** (Ed.) Penelope Hall's Social Services of England and Wales.
About 324 pp.
Morris, Mary. Voluntary Work and the Welfare State. *300 pp.*
Nokes, P. L. The Professional Task in Welfare Practice. *152 pp.*
Timms, Noel. Psychiatric Social Work in Great Britain (1939-1962).
280 pp.
●   Social Casework: *Principles and Practice. 256 pp.*
Young, A. F. Social Services in British Industry. *272 pp.*

SOCIOLOGY OF EDUCATION

Banks, Olive. Parity and Prestige in English Secondary Education: a Study in Educational Sociology. *272 pp.*

Bentwich, Joseph. Education in Israel. *224 pp. 8 pp. plates.*

●**Blyth, W. A. L.** English Primary Education. *A Sociological Description.*
   1. Schools. *232 pp.*
   2. Background. *168 pp.*

Collier, K. G. The Social Purposes of Education: *Personal and Social Values in Education. 268 pp.*

Dale, R. R., and **Griffith, S.** Down Stream: *Failure in the Grammar School. 108 pp.*

Evans, K. M. Sociometry and Education. *158 pp.*

●**Ford, Julienne.** Social Class and the Comprehensive School. *192 pp.*

Foster, P. J. Education and Social Change in Ghana. *336 pp. 3 maps.*

Fraser, W. R. Education and Society in Modern France. *150 pp.*

Grace, Gerald R. Role Conflict and the Teacher. *150 pp.*

Hans, Nicholas. New Trends in Education in the Eighteenth Century. *278 pp. 19 tables.*

● Comparative Education: *A Study of Educational Factors and Traditions. 360 pp.*

●**Hargreaves, David.** Interpersonal Relations and Education. *432 pp.*

● Social Relations in a Secondary School. *240 pp.*

Holmes, Brian. Problems in Education. *A Comparative Approach. 336 pp.*

King, Ronald. Values and Involvement in a Grammar School. *164 pp.*
   School Organization and Pupil Involvement. *A Study of Secondary Schools.*

●**Mannheim, Karl,** and **Stewart, W. A. C.** An Introduction to the Sociology of Education. *206 pp.*

Morris, Raymond N. The Sixth Form and College Entrance. *231 pp.*

●**Musgrove, F.** Youth and the Social Order. *176 pp.*

●**Ottaway, A. K. C.** Education and Society: An Introduction to the Sociology of Education. *With an Introduction by W. O. Lester Smith. 212 pp.*

Peers, Robert. Adult Education: *A Comparative Study. 398 pp.*

Pritchard, D. G. Education and the Handicapped: *1760 to 1960. 258 pp.*

Stratta, Erica. The Education of Borstal Boys. *A Study of their Educational Experiences prior to, and during, Borstal Training. 256 pp.*

Taylor, P. H., Reid, W. A., and **Holley, B. J.** The English Sixth Form. *A Case Study in Curriculum Research. 200 pp.*

SOCIOLOGY OF CULTURE

Eppel, E. M., and **M.** Adolescents and Morality: *A Study of some Moral Values and Dilemmas of Working Adolescents in the Context of a changing Climate of Opinion. Foreword by W. J. H. Sprott. 268 pp. 39 tables.*

●**Fromm, Erich.** The Fear of Freedom. *286 pp.*

● The Sane Society. *400 pp.*

Mannheim, Karl. Essays on the Sociology of Culture. *Edited by Ernst Mannheim in co-operation with Paul Kecskemeti. Editorial Note by Adolph Lowe. 280 pp.*

Weber, Alfred. Farewell to European History: *or The Conquest of Nihilism. Translated from the German by R. F. C. Hull. 224 pp.*

SOCIOLOGY OF RELIGION

Argyle, Michael and **Beit-Hallahmi, Benjamin.** The Social Psychology of Religion. *About 256 pp.*

Glasner, Peter E. The Sociology of Secularisation. *A Critique of a Concept. About 180 pp.*

Nelson, G. K. Spiritualism and Society. *313 pp.*

Stark, Werner. The Sociology of Religion. *A Study of Christendom.*
Volume I. *Established Religion. 248 pp.*
Volume II. *Sectarian Religion. 368 pp.*
Volume III. *The Universal Church. 464 pp.*
Volume IV. *Types of Religious Man. 352 pp.*
Volume V. *Types of Religious Culture. 464 pp.*

Turner, B. S. Weber and Islam. *216 pp.*

Watt, W. Montgomery. Islam and the Integration of Society. *320 pp.*

SOCIOLOGY OF ART AND LITERATURE

Jarvie, Ian C. Towards a Sociology of the Cinema. *A Comparative Essay on the Structure and Functioning of a Major Entertainment Industry. 405 pp.*

Rust, Frances S. Dance in Society. *An Analysis of the Relationships between the Social Dance and Society in England from the Middle Ages to the Present Day. 256 pp. 8 pp. of plates.*

Schücking, L. L. The Sociology of Literary Taste. *112 pp.*

Wolff, Janet. Hermeneutic Philosophy and the Sociology of Art. *150 pp.*

SOCIOLOGY OF KNOWLEDGE

Diesing, P. Patterns of Discovery in the Social Sciences. *262 pp.*

●**Douglas, J. D.** (Ed.) Understanding Everyday Life. *370 pp.*

●**Hamilton, P.** Knowledge and Social Structure. *174 pp.*

Jarvie, I. C. Concepts and Society. *232 pp.*

Mannheim, Karl. Essays on the Sociology of Knowledge. *Edited by Paul Kecskemeti. Editorial Note by Adolph Lowe. 353 pp.*

Remmling, Gunter W. The Sociology of Karl Mannheim. *With a Bibliographical Guide to the Sociology of Knowledge, Ideological Analysis, and Social Planning. 255 pp.*

Remmling, Gunter W. (Ed.) Towards the Sociology of Knowledge. *Origin and Development of a Sociological Thought Style. 463 pp.*

Stark, Werner. The Sociology of Knowledge: *An Essay in Aid of a Deeper Understanding of the History of Ideas. 384 pp.*

URBAN SOCIOLOGY

Ashworth, William. The Genesis of Modern British Town Planning: *A Study in Economic and Social History of the Nineteenth and Twentieth Centuries. 288 pp.*

Cullingworth, J. B. Housing Needs and Planning Policy: *A Restatement of the Problems of Housing Need and 'Overspill' in England and Wales. 232 pp. 44 tables. 8 maps.*

Dickinson, Robert E. City and Region: *A Geographical Interpretation 608 pp. 125 figures.*

The West European City: *A Geographical Interpretation. 600 pp. 129 maps. 29 plates.*

● The City Region in Western Europe. *320 pp. Maps.*

Humphreys, Alexander J. New Dubliners: *Urbanization and the Irish Family. Foreword by George C. Homans. 304 pp.*

Jackson, Brian. Working Class Community: *Some General Notions raised by a Series of Studies in Northern England. 192 pp.*

Jennings, Hilda. Societies in the Making: *a Study of Development and Redevelopment within a County Borough. Foreword by D. A. Clark. 286 pp.*

●**Mann, P. H.** An Approach to Urban Sociology. *240 pp.*

Morris, R. N., and **Mogey, J.** The Sociology of Housing. *Studies at Berinsfield. 232 pp. 4 pp. plates.*

Rosser, C., and **Harris, C.** The Family and Social Change. *A Study of Family and Kinship in a South Wales Town. 352 pp. 8 maps.*

●**Stacey, Margaret, Batsone, Eric, Bell, Colin,** and **Thurcott, Anne.** Power, Persistence and Change. *A Second Study of Banbury. 196 pp.*

RURAL SOCIOLOGY

Haswell, M. R. The Economics of Development in Village India. *120 pp.*

Littlejohn, James. Westrigg: *the Sociology of a Cheviot Parish. 172 pp. 5 figures.*

Mayer, Adrian C. Peasants in the Pacific. *A Study of Fiji Indian Rural Society. 248 pp. 20 plates.*

Williams, W. M. The Sociology of an English Village: *Gosforth. 272 pp. 12 figures. 13 tables.*

SOCIOLOGY OF INDUSTRY AND DISTRIBUTION

Anderson, Nels. Work and Leisure. *280 pp.*

●**Blau, Peter M.**, and **Scott, W. Richard.** Formal Organizations: *a Comparative approach. Introduction and Additional Bibliography by J. H. Smith. 326 pp.*

Dunkerley, David. The Foreman. *Aspects of Task and Structure. 192 pp.*

Eldridge, J. E. T. Industrial Disputes. *Essays in the Sociology of Industrial Relations. 288 pp.*

Hetzler, Stanley. Applied Measures for Promoting Technological Growth. *352 pp.*
Technological Growth and Social Change. *Achieving Modernization. 269 pp.*

Hollowell, Peter G. The Lorry Driver. *272 pp.*

●**Oxaal, I., Barnett, T.,** and **Booth, D.** (Eds). Beyond the Sociology of Development. *Economy and Society in Latin America and Africa. 295 pp.*

Smelser, Neil J. Social Change in the Industrial Revolution: *An Application of Theory to the Lancashire Cotton Industry, 1770–1840. 468 pp. 12 figures. 14 tables.*

ANTHROPOLOGY

Ammar, Hamed. Growing up in an Egyptian Village: *Silwa, Province of Aswan. 336 pp.*

Brandel-Syrier, Mia. Reeftown Elite. *A Study of Social Mobility in a Modern African Community on the Reef. 376 pp.*

Dickie-Clark, H. F. The Marginal Situation. *A Sociological Study of a Coloured Group. 236 pp.*

Dube, S. C. Indian Village. *Foreword by Morris Edward Opler. 276 pp. 4 plates.*
India's Changing Villages: *Human Factors in Community Development. 260 pp. 8 plates. 1 map.*

Firth, Raymond. Malay Fishermen. *Their Peasant Economy. 420 pp. 17 pp. plates.*

Gulliver, P. H. Social Control in an African Society: a Study of the Arusha, Agricultural Masai of Northern Tanganyika. *320 pp. 8 plates. 10 figures.*
Family Herds. *288 pp.*

Ishwaran, K. Tradition and Economy in Village India: *An Interactionist Approach. Foreword by Conrad Arensburg. 176 pp.*

Jarvie, Ian C. The Revolution in Anthropology. *268 pp.*

Little, Kenneth L. Mende of Sierra Leone. *308 pp. and folder.*
Negroes in Britain. *With a New Introduction and Contemporary Study by Leonard Bloom. 320 pp.*

Lowie, Robert H. Social Organization. *494 pp.*

Mayer, A. C. Peasants in the Pacific. *A Study of Fiji Indian Rural Society. 248 pp.*

Meer, Fatima. Race and Suicide in South Africa. *325 pp.*

Smith, Raymond T. The Negro Family in British Guiana: *Family Structure and Social Status in the Villages. With a Foreword by Meyer Fortes. 314 pp. 8 plates. 1 figure. 4 maps.*

Smooha, Sammy. Israel: Pluralism and Conflict. *About 320 pp.*

SOCIOLOGY AND PHILOSOPHY

Barnsley, John H. The Social Reality of Ethics. *A Comparative Analysis of Moral Codes. 448 pp.*

Diesing, Paul. Patterns of Discovery in the Social Sciences. *362 pp.*

●**Douglas, Jack D.** (Ed.) Understanding Everyday Life. *Toward the Recon- struction of Sociological Knowledge. Contributions by Alan F. Blum. Aaron W. Cicourel, Norman K. Denzin, Jack D. Douglas, John Heeren, Peter McHugh, Peter K. Manning, Melvin Power, Matthew Speier, Roy Turner, D. Lawrence Wieder, Thomas P. Wilson and Don H. Zimmerman. 370 pp.*

Gorman, Robert A. The Dual Vision. *Alfred Schutz and the Myth of Phenomenological Social Science. About 300 pp.*

Jarvie, Ian C. Concepts and Society. *216 pp.*

●**Pelz, Werner.** The Scope of Understanding in Sociology. *Towards a more radical reorientation in the social humanistic sciences. 283 pp.*

Roche, Maurice. Phenomenology, Language and the Social Sciences. *371 pp.*

Sahay, Arun. Sociological Analysis. *212 pp.*

Sklair, Leslie. The Sociology of Progress. *320 pp.*

Slater, P. Origin and Significance of the Frankfurt School. *A Marxist Perspective. About 192 pp.*

Smart, Barry. Sociology, Phenomenology and Marxian Analysis. *A Critical Discussion of the Theory and Practice of a Science of Society. 220 pp.*

International Library of Anthropology

General Editor Adam Kuper

Ahmed, A. S. Millenium and Charisma Among Pathans. *A Critical Essay in Social Anthropology. 192 pp.*

Brown, Paula. The Chimbu. *A Study of Change in the New Guinea High- lands. 151 pp.*

Gudeman, Stephen. Relationships, Residence and the Individual. *A Rural Panamanian Community. 288 pp. 11 Plates, 5 Figures, 2 Maps, 10 Tables.*

Hamnett, Ian. Chieftainship and Legitimacy. *An Anthropological Study of Executive Law in Lesotho. 163 pp.*

Hanson, F. Allan. Meaning in Culture. *127 pp.*

Lloyd, P. C. Power and Independence. *Urban Africans' Perception of Social Inequality. 264 pp.*

Pettigrew, Joyce. Robber Noblemen. *A Study of the Political System of the Sikh Jats. 284 pp.*

Street, Brian V. The Savage in Literature. *Representations of 'Primitive' Society in English Fiction, 1858–1920. 207 pp.*

Van Den Berghe, Pierre L. Power and Privilege at an African University. *278 pp.*

International Library of Social Policy

General Editor Kathleen Jones

Bayley, M. Mental Handicap and Community Care. *426 pp.*

Bottoms, A. E., and McClean, J. D. Defendants in the Criminal Process. *284 pp.*

Butler, J. R. Family Doctors and Public Policy. *208 pp.*

Davies, Martin. Prisoners of Society. *Attitudes and Aftercare. 204 pp.*

Gittus, Elizabeth. Flats, Families and the Under-Fives. *285 pp.*

Holman, Robert. Trading in Children. *A Study of Private Fostering. 355 pp.*

Jones, Howard, and Cornes, Paul. Open Prisons. *About 248 pp.*

Jones, Kathleen. History of the Mental Health Service. *428 pp.*

Jones, Kathleen, with Brown, John, Cunningham, W. J., Roberts, Julian, and Williams, Peter. Opening the Door. *A Study of New Policies for the Mentally Handicapped. 278 pp.*

Karn, Valerie. Retiring to the Seaside. *About 280 pp. 2 maps. Numerous tables.*

Thomas, J. E. The English Prison Officer since 1850: *A Study in Conflict. 258 pp.*

Walton, R. G. Women in Social Work. *303 pp.*

Woodward, J. To Do the Sick No Harm. *A Study of the British Voluntary Hospital System to 1875. 221 pp.*

International Library of Welfare and Philosophy

General Editors Noel Timms and David Watson

● **Plant, Raymond.** Community and Ideology. *104 pp.*

● **McDermott, F. E.** (Ed.) Self-Determination in Social Work. *A Collection of Essays on Self-determination and Related Concepts by Philosophers and Social Work Theorists. Contributors: F. P. Biestek, S. Bernstein, A. Keith-Lucas, D. Sayer, H. H. Perelman, C. Whittington, R. F. Stalley, F. E. McDermott, I. Berlin, H. J. McCloskey, H. L. A. Hart, J. Wilson, A. I. Melden, S. I. Benn. 254 pp.*

Ragg, Nicholas M. People Not Cases. *A Philosophical Approach to Social Work. About 250 pp.*

● **Timms, Noel,** and **Watson, David** (Eds). Talking About Welfare. *Readings in Philosophy and Social Policy. Contributors: T. H. Marshall, R. B. Brandt, G. H. von Wright, K. Nielsen, M. Cranston, R. M. Titmuss, R. S. Downie, E. Telfer, D. Donnison, J. Benson, P. Leonard, A. Keith-Lucas, D. Walsh, I. T. Ramsey. 320 pp.*

Primary Socialization, Language and Education

General Editor Basil Bernstein

Adlam, Diana S., *with the assistance of Geoffrey Turner and Lesley Lineker.* Code in Context. *About 272 pp.*

Bernstein, Basil. Class, Codes and Control. *3 volumes.*
 1. *Theoretical Studies Towards a Sociology of Language. 254 pp.*
 2. *Applied Studies Towards a Sociology of Language. 377 pp.*
 ● 3. *Towards a Theory of Educatiomal Transmission. 167 pp.*

Brandis, W., and **Bernstein, B.** Selection and Control. *176 pp.*

Brandis, Walter, and **Henderson, Dorothy.** Social Class, Language and Communication. *288 pp.*

Cook-Gumperz, Jenny. Social Control and Socialization. *A Study of Class Differences in the Language of Maternal Control. 290 pp.*

●**Gahagan, D. M.,** and **G. A.** Talk Reform. *Exploration in Language for Infant School Children. 160 pp.*

Hawkins, P. R. Social Class, the Nominal Group and Verbal Strategies. *About 220 pp.*

Robinson, W. P., and **Rackstraw, Susan D. A.** A Question of Answers. *2 volumes. 192 pp. and 180 pp.*

Turner, Geoffrey J., and **Mohan, Bernard A.** A Linguistic Description and Computer Programme for Children's Speech. *208 pp.*

Reports of the Institute of Community Studies

●**Cartwright, Ann.** Parents and Family Planning Services. *306 pp.*
 Patients and their Doctors. *A Study of General Practice. 304 pp.*

Dench, Geoff. Maltese in London. *A Case-study in the Erosion of Ethnic Consciousness. 302 pp.*

●**Jackson, Brian.** Streaming: *an Education System in Miniature. 168 pp.*

Jackson, Brian, and **Marsden, Dennis.** Education and the Working Class: *Some General Themes raised by a Study of 88 Working-class Children in a Northern Industrial City. 268 pp. 2 folders.*

Marris, Peter. The Experience of Higher Education. *232 pp. 27 tables.*
 Loss and Change. *192 pp.*

Marris, Peter, and **Rein, Martin.** Dilemmas of Social Reform. *Poverty and Community Action in the United States. 256 pp.*

Marris, Peter, and Somerset, Anthony. African Businessmen. *A Study of Entrepreneurship and Development in Kenya. 256 pp.*

Mills, Richard. Young Outsiders: *a Study in Alternative Communities. 216 pp.*

Runciman, W. G. Relative Deprivation and Social Justice. *A Study of Attitudes to Social Inequality in Twentieth-Century England. 352 pp.*

Willmott, Peter. Adolescent Boys in East London. *230 pp.*

Willmott, Peter, and Young, Michael. Family and Class in a London Suburb. *202 pp. 47 tables.*

Young, Michael. Innovation and Research in Education. *192 pp.*

●Young, Michael, and McGeeney, Patrick. Learning Begins at Home. *A Study of a Junior School and its Parents. 128 pp.*

Young, Michael, and Willmott, Peter. Family and Kinship in East London. *Foreword by Richard M. Titmuss. 252 pp. 39 tables.*

The Symmetrical Family. *410 pp.*

Reports of the Institute for Social Studies in Medical Care

Cartwright, Ann, Hockey, Lisbeth, and Anderson, John L. Life Before Death. *310 pp.*

Dunnell, Karen, and Cartwright, Ann. Medicine Takers, Prescribers and Hoarders. *190 pp.*

Medicine, Illness and Society

General Editor W. M. Williams

Robinson, David. The Process of Becoming Ill. *142 pp.*

Stacey, Margaret, *et al.* Hospitals, Children and Their Families. *The Report of a Pilot Study. 202 pp.*

Stimson, G. V., and Webb, B. Going to See the Doctor. *The Consultation Process in General Practice. 155 pp.*

Monographs in Social Theory

General Editor Arthur Brittan

●Barnes, B. Scientific Knowledge and Sociological Theory. *192 pp.*

Bauman, Zygmunt. Culture as Praxis. *204 pp.*

●Dixon, Keith. Sociological Theory. *Pretence and Possibility. 142 pp.*

Meltzer, B. N., Petras, J. W., and Reynolds, L. T. Symbolic Interactionism. *Genesis, Varieties and Criticisms. 144 pp.*

●Smith, Anthony D. The Concept of Social Change. *A Critique of the Functionalist Theory of Social Change. 208 pp.*

Routledge Social Science Journals

The British Journal of Sociology. *Editor – Angus Stewart; Associate Editor – Leslie Sklair. Vol. 1, No. 1 – March 1950 and Quarterly. Roy. 8vo. All back issues available. An international journal publishing original papers in the field of sociology and related areas.*

Community Work. *Edited by David Jones and Marjorie Mayo. 1973. Published annually.*

Economy and Society. *Vol. 1, No. 1. February 1972 and Quarterly. Metric Roy. 8vo. A journal for all social scientists covering sociology, philosophy, anthropology, economics and history. All back numbers available.*

Religion. Journal of Religion and Religions. *Chairman of Editorial Board, Ninian Smart. Vol. 1, No. 1, Spring 1971. A journal with an interdisciplinary approach to the study of the phenomena of religion. All back numbers available.*

Year Book of Social Policy in Britain, The. *Edited by Kathleen Jones. 1971. Published annually.*

Social and Psychological Aspects of Medical Practice

Editor Trevor Silverstone

Lader, Malcolm. Psychophysiology of Mental Illness. *280 pp.*

● **Silverstone, Trevor, and Turner, Paul.** Drug Treatment in Psychiatry. *232 pp.*

Printed in Great Britain by
Lowe & Brydone Printers Limited, Thetford, Norfolk